Before The Letdown: Dysphoric Milk Ejection Reflex And The Breastfeeding Mother

By Alia Macrina Heise, IBCLC

With an introduction by Diane Wiessinger, MS, IBCLC

Edited by Marcelina Watkinson, DClinPsy

Before The Letdown:
Dysphoric Milk Ejection Reflex (D-MER) And The Breastfeeding Mother
By Alia Macrina Heise, IBCLC

Table Of Contents

Preface

You've tried explaining your problem, and you do get answers:

"You just need to see a therapist. It sounds like postpartum depression." But almost all the time, you feel fine! "It's just baby blues." But multiple times a day, for a couple of minutes each time, you could almost kill yourself! Baby blues aren't that intense. "It's just your hormones. Give it some time." But it's been four months now! "Just put your baby on a bottle." But that's not at all what you want!

Or maybe, despite the horrid feelings that descend on you multiple times a day and then vanish like mist, you don't tell anyone at all, knowing you'll get one of those responses.

Even the word "just" in their responses belittles your experience and implies that there's a simple, one-step answer. Anywhere you turn, it seems, you come back misunderstood, dismissed, or alone.

Maybe what you're experiencing is D-MER – Dysphoric Milk Ejection Reflex. Typical symptoms are an abrupt change of mood when your milk releases. You may suddenly feel like the worst person on earth. Or you may feel nauseated, or confused. In its worst form, you may feel almost suicidal. In its mildest you may feel wistful or homesick. And then it lifts. Everything is as it was, and you feel like yourself. It's almost like a knee-jerk reaction. Once the feeling starts, there's no way to head it off. But it never lasts.

If anything in that description resonates with you, the insights and stories in this book can help. It was written because the book's lead author, Alia Heise, found herself with those symptoms and couldn't take "just" for an answer.

I'm one of the lactation consultants from whom Alia sought help early on. I suggested that it was probably a form of depression and she might want to talk to her doctor about it. (Not a helpful response, but I hope I didn't use the word "just"!) It was only when she contacted me again a few months later that I listened and learned and joined her in the early stages of her search for answers to a problem that didn't even have a name until she named it.

Alia created the d-mer.org website to connect mothers who experienced D-MER and was stunned by the rapid and sizeable response. They learned from her, and she learned from them. She, several lactation consultants, and a medical school student formed a "think tank" to try to sort out D-MER's triggers and infer from them what the physiology might be. Alia was both leader and guinea-pig-in-chief. As her book explains, we finally settled on dopamine, or rather a lack of dopamine, as a likely culprit. And that led to insights into limiting and even eliminating symptoms. In my thirty-some years as a breastfeeding helper and specialist, I think being involved in those early D-MER investigations was one of the most important things I accomplished. For me it was a fascinating experience. For Alia it has become a life's work.

In this book, and on the website d-mer.org, you'll learn that you're part of a sizeable club. How sizeable? That's one of the many things we don't know. D-MER isn't a common

7

experience, and it has been virtually invisible until very recently. Maybe in part because, for decades and even today, breastfeeding a baby wasn't/isn't seen as a truly normal part of life in the first place. Any glitches in this already-questionable system were... well, just (there's that word again) one of those things. Not anymore.

What we are certain of at this point is that mothers with D-MER deserve a way to connect with one another. The website d-mer.org can give you that connection. And mothers with D-MER deserve all the information that has accumulated so far. This book can give you that.

In these pages are mothers' stories, thoughts on the mechanism involved, descriptions of D-MER's several forms, ways to cope, and concrete suggestions that may reduce or even eliminate your symptoms. You're not crazy, you're not the only one, and you're not without resources.

Our strong hunch – that a temporary and too-deep drop in dopamine occurs for some women when their milk releases – is still just a hunch. We badly need research to confirm or refute that hunch so that we can move to faster and better help from our healthcare providers, better-targeted solutions, and better understanding and support among our friends and family.

You can help. Do you know – or know someone who knows – a researcher in neuroscience or endocrinology who might add a piece to the puzzle? Do you know a breastfeeding counselor or specialist in maternity care who would benefit from the information? Pass on this book and the Heise/

8

Wiessinger article in International Breastfeeding Journal (google D-MER International Breastfeeding Journal). Together, we can ensure that the second edition of this book offers even more and better help.

In the meantime, you can help by sharing your own story and resources, on the website, with friends, with your healthcare team. You're not "just" another case. If you experience D-MER and are looking for answers, you are one of a tribe of women making their way through this tangled part of the motherhood maze with curiosity and courage. You're smoothing the path for mothers yet to come. And we thank you.

Diane Wiessinger, MS, IBCLC
December, 2017

Introduction
This is a book for mothers and for breastfeeding supporters and helpers alike. There is not a lot known or understood about dysphoric milk ejection reflex, but what is known and understood, as well as what is estimated and hypothesized, is the information brought together here. The knowledge, anecdotes, suggestions and stories about D-MER have been spread throughout cyber space; and now, unlike in 2007, they can easily be found through a Google search. But this book will be the first attempt to consolidate the information on a topic that has been discussed openly now, with maternal and professional recognition, for 10 years. And yet, there is still no evidenced based research on D-MER to reference or speak to. It is an incredibly under researched complaint that needs and deserves more attention. That does not mean,

however, that D-MER has any less impact on mothers, or any less credence to the experience of the breastfeeding dyad. The one thing that cannot be refuted, is that hundreds and hundreds of mothers have come forward and joined together in an online presence to find understanding and camaraderie in their seemingly strange and unique emotional ordeal of the milk ejection reflex. Through this book there will be clarification of what D-MER is, what it is not, how D-MER presents and the patterns seen between women, thoughts on the future of understanding D-MER better, how to help and support mothers through their trials, as well as quotes and stories from mothers themselves.

*Throughout this writing I use the word "mother" and the pronoun "she" for simplicity of language. This is not to exclude any breastfeeding trans-male parents or to exclude anyone who refers to themselves in a different pronoun. Thank you for your understanding.

**As the author, I am an International Board Certified Lactation Consultant. I am not a doctor, a general health care provider or a medical professional that is able to give medical advice. It is not in my scope of practice to suggest treatments, solutions, herbs or medications to mothers. The appropriate health care professional needs to be consulted if a mother decides to pursue these kinds of solutions for her D-MER. Also, there is not yet any evidenced based information about D-MER. All information in this book has been collected from pattern observation and information gathering from mothers who have self-reported that they have D-MER.

*** *It is worth noting that the use of the word "condition" and "diagnosis" has been deliberately avoided in the writing of this information, whenever possible. This is because it is not known how rare or how common D-MER is. It may be very much in the spectrum of a normal, albeit uncomfortable, breastfeeding occurrence. Though there are extreme cases where intervention to correct or ease D-MER are called for so that a mother and baby can continue their breastfeeding journey, the majority of mothers find enough comfort in information and peer support to continue breastfeeding without medical treatment. Some mothers find a sense of ease in having a "diagnosis" of a "condition" for D-MER. Having the terms, labels and names can be an empowering and validating part of their journey. It allows them to let go of the idea of being crazy or abnormal, it can enable them to speak more confidently about their circumstance and it gives them a tool for talking to medical professionals. On the other side of the coin, some mothers feel that a diagnosis can pathologize and shame the mother, as diagnoses have a way of suggesting a defect within the individual. A diagnosis also misses the importance of context and the wider picture, and can make someone feel like they have no power to influence the outcome. Another perspective is that some mothers prefer to see their experience as just another version of normality, finding a lack of diagnostic labeling to be more freeing and without stigma or shame. There is no one right way or one answer for this, though in a society of jargon and acronyms, it is not surprising that more often than not, it is more common for D-MER to be referenced as a breastfeeding condition.*

**** *The quotes included in the book were taken from various places including surveys, questionnaires, the D-MER.org website and the D-MER Facebook support group. Permission was asked wherever possible. Identifying information has been removed for the mother's privacy.*

Chapter One
The Story Behind D-MER

In 2007, the year my third child was born, there was not such a term as "dysphoric milk ejection reflex". All there was, were a handful of threads on the mothering.com forum with a few brave and struggling breastfeeding mothers saying, "I feel like emotional sewage when I breastfeed my baby". As you can imagine, this is not the most popular phase to utter inside any strongly pro-breastfeeding circles. Breastfeeding is something that is still held in high regard as an overwhelmingly positive choice, experience and decision. It is touted as being something that is bonding, that creates warm and fuzzy feelings and is a beautiful madonna-esque experience. But thanks to the bravery of the moms that initially spoke up about a seemingly shameful challenge, one different than the usual early days of sore nipples, there are now hundreds of women who continue to speak up and who have found help, peace of mind and answers from the awareness that has arisen about an issue that is now call dysphoric milk ejection reflex.

If there is anything I have learned from being in the field of lactation for 11 years, it is that every breastfeeding issue is enlightened by a story. We all have a story to tell and D-MER mothers have a unique experience and immense challenges and are in desperate need of a voice and recognition for their struggles and situation. They have a desire to tell their story, and to have it validated by the stories of other D-MER mothers.

So it makes sense to begin with the story of the birth of the term dysphoric milk ejection reflex, which came shortly after the birth of my third baby.

In 2007 I had been working in the field of lactation for over 3 years. I had started out as a trained peer counselor, and by the time I was expecting my third child, I was a Certified Lactation Counselor (CLC). I had had two previous breastfeeding experiences with my first two children, each with their own individual, but not unique, challenges. I had a culmination of nearly three years of not only personal breastfeeding experience, but also of professional experience in my work with other breastfeeding mothers, through two different organizations. Having had a medicated and intervention filled vaginal hospital delivery with my first, and a natural hospital delivery with my second, I had planned and prepared for a home birth for my third.

I successfully had a perfectly planned homebirth for my third child, a daughter, named Elliotte. The birth itself was only unique in the fact that it was precipitous. There were no interventions other than blue cohosh and caster oil to initially stimulate labor due to leaking amniotic fluid after my due date. There was also no separation of mother and baby at any time. I had nursed my previous two children a combined 29 months without any problems, and planned to do the same with this child. I had a very relaxing postpartum period with lots of support from family and friends. But fairly soon into this postpartum period I began feeling a frequent "yuckyness." I had nothing to connect it to. It was sporadic. I figured maybe it was just the coming and going of baby blues, though I had no prior history with depression, postpartum depression (PPD) or otherwise.

A few weeks further in, I decided I needed to look into my waves of negative emotion more and continued to considered that it was possibly just postpartum depression, but I felt that it was unlikely and the idea did not sit quite right. Because of my support system and the nature of my birth and postpartum period I knew I was in a low risk category for depression. But something was "off."

What I was experiencing, about 10-15 times a day, was a sickening hollow feeling in the pit of my stomach. There would be a strong aversion to food. I would not feel sad per say, but I would feel "icky and yucky" and pretty hopeless and melancholy with lots of shame and feelings of worthlessness and uncertainty. I sometimes would feel down right suicidal for a passing moment. It was a highly negative emotional state to feel. It was a feeling I seemed to have associated with strong feelings of worry and guilt in the past, because when I first started experiencing the sensation I kept searching for what I was feeling guilty or worried about. It always turned out there was nothing; it was just that same sinking feeling in the pit of my stomach that I had must have experienced in the past for some reason. It would last for about one to two minutes every time, which sounds very brief, but it was so overwhelming that it would grab my attention from nearly anything I was doing. It was so concerning and derailing that as I try to catch up to it, I would end up needing to focus my way through it, nearly like I needed to for a contraction during labor. The rest of the day I would be fine, in fact often I was great.

As I was perusing online forums for PPD to get a grasp of what was happening, there was a thread entitled "Only When Nursing." I saw it day after day and never looked at it. After all, what I was feeling was not only when nursing, it was sometimes when my baby was not at the breast. Finally I decided to click on it and read it; I figured that as least because I was a lactation counselor it would be a good thing to learn about. A low mood only when nursing was nothing I had ever learned about in all my training and though the forum was not of a professional nature, if there were moms experiencing it, I figured I should learn about their experiences. So I opened the thread and read about dozens of other woman describing the exact same feelings and timing that I had been having, most of them never having talked about it until then. But for these women it was connected to breastfeeding. I had never made that connection for myself. Then I realized that in my case it was related to letdown, which for me, happened not only when breastfeeding, but many times throughout the day in-between nursing as well. I had an abundant milk supply and my breasts would often release milk due to over fullness. With this in mind, I started noticing that it was about 30 seconds before my milk letdown, this intense emotional letdown happened, too. It was indeed connected to lactation after all. It was amazing to hear the words of these women online explaining with their own words the exact same bizarre feelings I had been having. But there seemed to be no identified cause. Many women just said, *"yes, that's me too, it's horrible"* or *"I thought I was all alone"* or *"it finally went away when I weaned; I could not take it any longer."* I was wondering, is there anyone who knows why we were all going through this nightmare every time our milk letdown?

After that information and knowing that I was at least not alone, I found that over a few weeks' time that just having the awareness of the feelings and knowing that it was not my job to fix them or address them, made a big difference. One thing I had taught myself was that it was not real. Very frequently when a letdown would hit I would be thinking about something specific: a purchase made, something I had said to my mother, an interaction I had with my husband, an email I had sent, anything. These thoughts could be very positive and wonderful things, but when the letdown hit me I suddenly was overcome with guilt, remorse, confusion and shame over whatever it was that I was thinking about. I would start trying to figure out why I was feeling bad all of a sudden; trying to link it to the specific thought. *"Was it an irresponsible purchase? Did I speak impulsively? Did I offend him? Should I have not blind copied that other recipient?"* The reaction to letdown would for some reason put anxiety and doubts into my mind - serious doubts that could even turn something fine or something wonderful, feel wrong. But as I finally realized these confused, worrisome feelings had nothing to do with the thoughts or issues and it was all about the letdown, things felt easier. These feelings were in fact unrelated and the worry that ensued was unfounded with no valid basis whatsoever. It was simply some kind of lactation hormonal related cause. So after

16

realizing that it was indeed somehow connected to lactation, when it hit I knew to clear my mind, or distract myself until it passed. I did not waste my time even trying to figure out if the guilt or remorse was valid or true or not. I just determine that it was all false and moved on.

Generally it was getting easier to handle as I was learning my own tricks for coping and was able to explain it away, but there were still these very hard times. It was the evening times that were still the hardest. That was when my little one wanted to nurse and nurse and nurse before falling asleep for the night. And I was alone in a dark room with nothing but my thoughts and feelings. I was supposed to be treasuring the snuggles and the quiet time and instead I was ready to run away screaming. Doubt about my own emotional reactions still existed and furthermore, as a breastfeeding counselor I was feeling very frustrated at the numbers of women suffering through, or weaning because of this problem. A problem that seemed to have no answer.

As I continued to scour the internet for information, I found that there were indeed lactation professionals that were coming across mothers that were reporting similar ailments. Finding this information was amazing. There were even more mothers out there like me, and there were lactation consultants that were inquiring about it. I scoured the online message board threads to find out what was being done about it. Included below are just a handful of posts from breastfeeding professionals about this phenomenon. The quotes are taken from a message board for lactation consultants (LC's). The posts range in timeline from 1998-2004.

A pediatrician has asked me about a 7-week mom who experiences depression with each milk release. The depression lifts after a few minutes. I found a bit in the archives, but am wondering about mechanism and treatment. Vasopressin (ADH or antidiuretic hormone) can be linked to depression. Does anyone know whether/how it's involved with oxytocin? Apparently the two are very similar chemically. Something somewhere makes me think there's a connection between the thirst that milk release generates and the fleeting depression this mom experiences. I've suggested that she use a good book, a good book on tape, or good music (all her definition of "good") to distract her during letdown, and that most likely the symptom will abate with time. I'm also wondering if just possibly drinking water during letdown might help. Why am I connecting the depression and the milk-release thirst? Does it make sense to anyone else?

I have been lurking for a while and now have a question. Today I had a patient, a pediatrician, who gave birth to her 4th baby 2 days ago. At the end of my shift she asked if she could speak to me privately. This mom breastfeeds her babies for a long time but since her 2nd birth she has had a disquieting phenomenon. As soon as her milk comes down she feels a feeling of sadness and aggressiveness. She cannot bear anyone to come near her, not even the children. This happens at each breastfeeding session for two or three weeks, and then disappears. She wanted to know if I had ever come across a woman with similar complaints. I had not. I could not explore this much further with her because she was on her way home, but I promised to throw this out to you all. Has anyone seen a woman with similar complaints? Would anyone have an explanation? She attributes it to "hormones" and although she assumes it is temporary, as in the past, she finds these feelings very uncomfortable.

* I am a LC with a question from a long distance friend. My history may be inadequate as this was very brief conversation. Anyway here goes: a second time mother has been experiencing depression only when her milk lets down, she is nursing her 3 week old infant and has been experiencing this "tearfulness" and, as she calls it "depression only when she nurses her baby". She experienced this with her first child as well, and weaned at 6 months, because of the sadness and tearfulness she was experiencing. Following the weaning of her 6 month old, the depression improved. She is considering weaning again because of this. I was unable to find anything in the literature I read. I do not have the luxury of asking her all the questions I would like to, but when I do ask, I want to ask the correct ones. Have any of you heard of this experience? She mentions she feels fine when she is not nursing. Could be some deep personal history, or perhaps a physiological explanation? Any insights are much appreciated.

* D wrote that a mum in her group mentioned prolactin during letdown causing anxiety, nervousness hyperactivity. I recall, with each of my three, just for the first week of breastfeeding, feeling a fleeting, but very profound, feeling of utter misery at letdown, lasting 1-3 seconds at most, a kind of going to the dentist/got an exam feeling, then

complete recovery. One other mother to whom I mentioned this, said she had a similar thing; she experienced fleeting anxiety.

* Several years I worked with a mother (who happened to be a clinical psychologist) who reported to me that she felt depressed each time she sat down to nurse and then the feeling would pass after a couple of minutes into the nursing. She would be fine until the next nursing. She was an avid nurser and the infant was nursing well. She had had no problems with depression before. She went on an extended out of town trip for a couple of months and when she returned she reported that she no longer had those depressed feelings; as I recall it seemed to go away at around the third month or so. I also had a mom who felt nausea with letdown and several who had headaches with letdown. All of this passed within a few months. These moms were persistent and they went on to enjoy symptom free nursings. The power of oxytocin?

*I am working with a mother of a three month old. This is her third child. She complains of extreme nausea when her milk lets down. But also "having all kinds of bad feeling churned up from her insides," feelings of destructiveness ("like I want to take this glass and smash it against the wall") and a general feeling of being dangerously out of control for those few moments at the start of a feeding. Then she realizes what it is, again, and gets a hold of herself. She assures me she would never act on these feelings. She had the same feelings with her first, now 3 years of age, but much milder. And with her second, now 18 months, but a bit stronger, so she was greatly relieved to

*quit breastfeeding that child when she became pregnant
with this third one. I discussed with her oxytocin release,
drinking more water each day, eating prior to
breastfeeding to control the nausea. Also ambivalence
about breastfeeding (she does feel ambivalent, but because
of the nausea and emotions, she says) and the possibility of
abuse in her history (she feels that is not a factor for her).
Two other things: mother and baby are dealing with yeast
and mother reports very strong letdowns and her milk
coming in even when she's not feeding the baby, but if it is
around feeding times, even at this late date of three months
postpartum. Any ideas? And if it is excessive levels of
oxytocin, is there any treatment you know of?*

These professionals were talking about it, but on one was
really doing anything about it. There were no clear responses
to any of these posts. Most were neglected completely. No
one had answers, there was no explanation, no help and at
this point in the story D-MER still did not even have a name.
Mainly, I was still working on my own to figure it out; which
was very limiting. Yes, I was coping better with my own
emotional challenges of D-MER myself, but I could not let go
of the fact that this was something that was happening to
other mothers, LC's were talking about it but no one was
truly recognizing it and there was no understanding brought
to it. I continued on tirelessly with my searches and after
weeks of digging and of trying all sorts of doors, I felt that I
had stumbled upon a lead that led somewhere. As I
abandoned my keyword searches and started tapping into
my own professional resources instead, I found a helpful
soul. This LC was not just anyone, either, but a renowned
breastfeeding "guru" that lived an hour away, someone I had

met, seen speak publicly, and even emailed with before. It was through the posts of lactation consultants casually seeking answers to this problem. Her post on the LC board about the depression/letdown problem had been years ago, but I emailed her on the off chance that she was still interested in figuring it out; and she was. This LC was one that was not dismissive but embraced her natural curiosity, took time for me and at least had some theories for me. Not only that, but she got two other lactation consultants, who were also published authors, involved in the email discussion with me.

All together we first discussed and ruled out this possibility given by one expert: *"...a mammal mother who eats or pushes away or kicks or otherwise abuses any baby that is not her own. Is it possible that these mothers are getting a negative feeling about the baby, but are so culturally/mentally committed to the baby that they do not make the connection? Might it be the flip side of oxytocin - an urge to get away from anyone who is not "your own"? Something drives the typical mammal mother to refuse to nurse the alien baby. Are these mothers picking up the scent of a strange baby? Could separation of mother and baby create a refusal response?"* However, I had an easy home birth with no separation from my baby and so based on my case alone we were able to rule out that theory as a problem in this case. Next came another idea from another lactation professional: *"Letdown triggers oxytocin, and high levels of oxytocin can trigger unremembered feelings of abuse. Since at least one third of women in North America were sexually abused, this is another possible cause of depression during letdown. When I worked as a doula, some very surprising memories sometimes surfaced during the transition phase of labor that the woman did not remember before or afterwards."* Agreeing that this could cause all sorts of breastfeeding problems in some cases, once again we ruled it out for this particular problem, as this was my third baby, but it was my first time with this problem. If it was repressed trauma, it would have affected me before. Additionally, with my experience it was not isolated to nipple contact by any means, it was connected to the milk ejection reflex (MER), whether I was breastfeeding at the time or not.

After these initial theories we explored so many more possibilities that I will not spend the time explaining them all in detail. But in short we explored, and ultimately tabled the idea of these following issues being the main culprit: oxytocin, prolactin, vasopressin, thyroid, pituitary gland, the amygdala, history of abuse, history of mental illness, medications used in labor, separation of mother and baby and more.... all of these before finally discovering that dopamine had a major role in lactation, a role not very well known or included in lactation education thus far, as it had not been an issue in the relatively new science of lactation before. However, when it came to D-MER, dopamine made sense.

I will share an initial blog post that I wrote once we first reached this part of the journey:

" I am giving something new a little look: dopamine. I started to think more about some people's dysphoric reaction (an unpleasant or uncomfortable mood, such as sadness, a depressed mood, anxiety, irritability, or

restlessness) to the drug metoclopramide (Reglan). The dysphoria this reaction causes is reminiscent of how it feels in comparison to some people's experience with D-MER. This includes my own sensitivity to Reglan and its similarity to D-MER feelings. I decided to investigate metoclopramide and it's mechanisms more.

Metoclopramide is also used as a galactagogue (a medication to increase milk supply) and it's general mechanism is to block dopamine receptors, it's a dopamine antagonist. When someone has a bad reaction to metoclopramide it can cause dysphoria, including suicidal ideation. This is may be because of the person's reaction to lack of dopamine, or because the metoclopramide is blocking too many receptors.

When metoclopramide is used in lactation, as a milk increaser, it is used because dopamine inhibits prolactin production. So by using metoclopramide, one will block the dopamine receptors, reducing the amount of dopamine that is in the body that is inhibiting prolactin secretion. Dopamine is the primary neuroendocrine inhibitor of the secretion of prolactin from the anterior pituitary gland. The lactotrope cells that produce prolactin, in the absence of dopamine, secrete prolactin continuously and dopamine inhibits this secretion. So, in the context of regulating prolactin secretion, dopamine is occasionally called prolactin-inhibiting factor (PIF), prolactin-inhibiting hormone (PIH), or prolactostatin. Prolactin also seems to inhibit dopamine release, such as after orgasm, and is chiefly responsible for the refractory period.

Dopamine has many functions in the brain, including important roles in behavior and cognition, motor activity, motivation and reward, inhibition of prolactin production (involved in lactation), sleep, mood, attention, and learning. Dopamine is commonly associated with the pleasure system of the brain, providing feelings of enjoyment and reinforcement to motivate a person proactively to perform certain activities. Dopamine is released by naturally rewarding experiences such as food, sex, some drugs, and neutral stimuli that become associated with them. Dopamine is at work in motor control areas in the brain as well as thinking areas of the brain.

From everything I have read it would be dopamine and its work within the thinking areas of the brain that would be pertinent. In that area dopamine is responsible for feelings of bliss and pleasure, euphoria, appetite control and feeling focused. If you take a quick look at the emotional symptoms of D-MER you have feelings of displeasure, dysphoria, loss of appetite and lack of focus.

It would not be truly possible for D-MER mothers to have low levels of dopamine all the time. There are too many reports of feeling good, even elated, in between letdowns. Interestingly as dopamine levels rise one becomes excited and energized. Too high though and it turns into paranoia and a feeling of over stimulation, a feeling I can sometimes attest to as well as the elevated and energized mood at times. If dopamine stays low it is associated with low mood, depression, poor concentration and memory and fatigue. So of course I am thinking that during a D-MER episode a mother may have inappropriately low levels of dopamine but it's not straight forward, this is where the hormonal milieu comes into play. It's not going to be "just" dopamine or "just" oxytocin; it's going to be "something" playing off of "something" when "something" is not right with this other "something!"

There is also the phenomenon of dysphoria, not just low mood, but also feelings of panic, anxiousness, irritability, restlessness, need to "get away" and suicidal ideation, when dopamine is suppressed by drugs. These are feelings dopamine is not usually held responsible for on its own, but feeling that are expressed within the context of D-MER.

One reason I started to get excited about the idea of dopamine is because I was finally able to connect that idea to other factors and questions that have come into play. 1.) One important connection here is that low levels of dopamine are connected very directly to restless leg syndrome (RLS). Several mothers who have experiences RSL syndrome have connected the emotional feeling of D-MER to the feeling during an RSL episode. 2.) Another connecting factor is that dopamine is released with cigarette smoking. And smoking, we have found out, diminished the feeling of D-MER within a certain time frame. 3.) Dopamine takes a big drop after orgasm and seems key in determining sexual satiety within its relationship to prolactin. Is this a start of an explanation for what some women experience post coital dysphoria (PCD?) 4.) High calorie foods increase dopamine, perhaps why a mother may not feel a D-MER after severely overeating?

26

That's a lot of information for now, and it answers no questions, but only asks more, but it is a very interesting angle to be discovering."

Shortly after beginning to work with some other lactation professionals I was also beginning to find more mothers with D-MER. The stories included those with mild symptoms, those who put it together once hearing about it, and those who had it disrupting their whole life. I had no way of determining the percentage of mothers that were encountering this. I had found nearing seventy-five mothers across only three forums within mere weeks. Most admitted they were too embarrassed to ever say anything to anyone before, which is probably one of the reasons D-MER had gone without proper attention all that time.

I was also finding myself disappointed and sometimes straight out angry with the lactation community. As a CLC at the time I took much pride in the lactation consultants worldwide and I had been proud to consider myself among them. But here was something many of them had gotten wind of some way or another and they had dismissed it, denied it and over looked it. In regards to this particular issue, I felt that the lactation community had failed the population of breastfeeding mothers. I was feeling vindicated that now they would no longer wonder why some women choose not to nurse because the mothers vaguely did not like breastfeeding, and they could no longer avoid educating pregnant and nursing mothers about such a pertinent issue. I was also encouraged that at least some of the lactation consultants were listening. This was emailed to me by one of the lactation consultants I was corresponding with: *"it seems to me one thing we can do for all of you is to acknowledge that this happens, that it's not terribly uncommon, that it often but by no means always goes away on its own, and that we're working to find a reason and solution. You're right; it's been swept under the table. No one likes to admit that something icky exists without explanation or solution. Better to say it's uncommon and will go away on its own and move on to something more fun, like breast abscesses. You're casting light into a dark corner, and it's time someone did!"* That was one of the most validating things I received at the time.

By the time my baby was a year old the team that I was working with and I had named the anomaly as dysphoric milk ejection reflex, several hundred mothers had been informally interviewed and D-MER was being accepted by lactation professionals as something that affected the breastfeeding mother, her experience and the duration of lactation for a baby. Our informal investigation into dopamine continued to be an appropriate guess, enough so that we felt comfortable putting it on the table as the most likely culprit for D-MER. After observing how D-MER was affected by nicotine, pseudoephedrine, over indulgence in chocolate and sugar, orgasm, certain herbal remedies and a couple prescription medications; the theory held and remains the current most plausible theory for D-MER at this time.

I nursed my baby until she self weaned at three and a half years. I continued to have D-MER until she was two and a half, but it did diminish in severity as time went on. I tried a variety of treatments and solutions, spending a good amount of time as a human guinea pig for D-MER. I did finally settle on an herb that did ease the intensity of D-MER for the last year or so. I had, what is known now as, a severe case of despondency D-MER and was subjected to urges to self injure and suicidal ideation when it was at it's worst. I had about six months of emotionally peaceful breastfeeding until I started experiencing nursing aversion during our last six months of nursing.

The emotional disturbance and trauma that I experienced with D-MER is now a vague memory, though the impact that the experience had on me, shaped me. Not only has it became my life's work and goal to continue to work with D-MER and make D-MER my niche in the field of my profession, but it also shaped me personally. D-MER challenged and extended my emotional intelligence and my self awareness. It played on my highly sensitive nature and empathic personality. It pointed me in the direction of mindfulness, forced me to better understand feelings of self shame and after it broke me, it allowed me to build myself back up. Not everyone may be able to look back on their time spent hand in hand and heart in heart with D-MER, and feel like it made a lifetime impact on their psyches. But I have no regrets for what life handed me when it handed me D-MER, and I have no doubt that the various personal details of my life, the ones from before and after D-MER, as well as the veracity of my D-MER itself, set me up to be the one to bring better understanding about D-MER to the field of lactation and to the mothers that it supports.

Chapter Two
What D-MER Is

The definition of D-MER stands alone as: dysphoric milk ejection reflex is a condition affecting lactating women that is characterized by an abrupt dysphoria, negative emotions, that occur just before milk release and continues for not more than a few minutes.

In further explanation, D-MER is triggered when the milk ejection reflex is triggered. The MER in a lactating mother can be triggered by suckling, overfilled breasts, sounds of her baby crying, and a variety of other possibilities. MERs can happen when breastfeeding or pumping, but can also be spontaneous and happen when not breastfeeding. A mother with D-MER will experience the dysphoria of D-MER whenever the MER is triggered, though the intensity of her dysphoric experience can vary.

Dysphoria with MER during breastfeeding is the criterion for identification and D-MER seems to have some key components and few variances between mothers. There are reoccurring phrases and words that mothers use to describe their experience, but the emotional colors that a mother may experience can vary between ranging from sadness and dread to anxiety to anger. These emotions fall on the D-MER spectrum which has three different intensities of mild, moderate and severe. A mother with D-MER experiences feelings that often manifest "in the mother's stomach" - a hollow feeling, a feeling like there is something in the pit of the stomach, or an emotional churning in the stomach.

The common thread between these three different emotional spectrums is the wave of negative emotions; the dysphoria, prior to letdown. This happens when nursing and most often with expressing and spontaneous letdowns as well. The dysphoria then lifts within another 30-90 seconds, and then usually repeats with each letdown.

A key piece of D-MER is that a mother with D-MER feels absolutely fine except just before her milk starts to flow. D-MER is a brief feeling, not more than 30 seconds to 2 minutes, only and always beginning before letdown. It is not postpartum depression and most mothers feel perfectly fine except for that pre-milk moment. A brief interval after the negative feelings appear, the milk begins to flow.

Tell Tale Manifestation Of D-MER
As previously mentioned, D-MER has some key components and few variances between mothers and it presents itself in some very distinct ways with some highly recognizable markers for almost all D-MER mothers (see figure 4).

- Mother's will note that the feelings come on suddenly, and dissipate within a short amount of time.
- The feelings are in conjunction with her milk releasing.
- The emotional reaction will be felt before she feels any physical sensation of letdown in her breasts.
- Many mothers explain an emotional manifestation that happens in her stomach or gut.
- Her feelings are generally self directed.

These are the key components of D-MER, there are some other notable trends and commonalities between mothers with D-MER that will be further explained and mentioned, but the above points are the attributes of D-MER that make it most distinctive and recognizable.

The Spectrums And Intensities Of D-MER

D-MER is currently categorized into three different spectrums and three different intensities. The spectrums are defined as despondency, anxiety and agitation. These spectrums are used to describe the mother's emotional experience with D-MER. The intensities are clarified as mild, moderate and severe and are used to explain the level of disturbance and extremeness of a mother's emotional interlude. There is a specificity in how these can manifest for a mother with D-MER. A mother with despondency D-MER can find herself with a mild, moderate or severe presentation. Though a mother with anxiety D-MER will see that her D-MER is either moderate or severe. Lastly, a mother with agitation D-MER will always report that her D-MER is severe. This rationally aligns with logic, as the spectrum of D-MER is a progression of what one would see with the explanation of the progression of intense emotions. Depression is a less aggressive sensation than anxiety and the aggression of agitation D-MER is a much more intense experience than depression or anxiety. This is not to say that depression is not intense, it is, and the intensity of a depressive feeling for the mother with severe despondency D-MER is quite serious. The progression is more the color or inward interpretation of the emotion. Sadness is blue and anger is red, is a good example. Another way to say it is that though one can feel severely depressed, it is rare that one says they are mildly angry. In this way, the D-MER spectrums and intensities seem to align (see figure 5).

Spectrums

Some mothers have more of a sad, depressive experience and therefor are have a case of the despondency spectrum of D-MER. One mother articulated, *"every time I sit down to feed I feel a rush of sadness to the depths of my soul, guilt, I want to cry my eyes out! I feel like my whole world is about to come crashing down"*. Despondency D-MER seems to be the most common experience among self-reporting mothers. Other mothers have more panicky, restless, or fearful feelings during the MER and these mother's would classify as being within the anxiety spectrum of D-MER. As a mother expressed, *"a let down brings a crashing wave of panic and anxiety. It just lasts for a few seconds (thank God), and it makes me feel completely crazy."* This spectrum is less common than despondency spectrum but occurs more often than the last spectrum, which is agitation D-MER. Mother's who fall into the agitation spectrum of D-MER struggle with feelings of irritation, anger or frustration (see figures 6-8). As a mother shared, *"I have heard a lot of you describe your experiences as overwhelming sadness, depression, emptiness etc. I was just wondering if anyone else ever feels overwhelming anger and rage which literally makes you want to smack your head against a brick wall and stop breathing. This is coupled with simultaneous guilt and self loathing and is so indescribably horrible that just writing about it gives me anxiety. If I'm being honest sometimes my anger is towards my little girl (although I would never take it out on her) until I remind myself that I am the issue, not*

33

her, then I hate myself even more. I feel like the worst mother and a horrible human being and to make it worse I feel like no one will listen to me or take me seriously. I feel so lost right now. I do not wish this upon my worst enemy but would like to know if there is anyone out there who feels this intense rage?" It has been noted that mother's exist within a single spectrum for the duration of breastfeeding with D-MER. Hence, a mother does not feel despondent at one feeding and agitated at another. The color and feel of the emotional reaction is consistent throughout her time struggling with D-MER.

Intensity

Next to be discussed is the intensity of the emotional experience. A mother will feel the negative emotional reaction of D-MER either mildly, moderately or severely. Mild D-MER is the most prevalent reported situation with severe D-MER being the least common. Mild D-MER tends to self-correct the soonest, tends to be the most tolerable and the least distressing and often mothers find that education about the particulars of their experience is the only treatment or solution needed to continue on with their breastfeeding journey. Mother's with severe D-MER are the ones who are more interested in any solutions or treatment that may be available to try, they are at the highest risk for weaning and even with education, they find D-MER to be a very invasive part of the breastfeeding journey. Mother's with moderate D-MER fall in-between these two presentations (see figures 9-12). The intensity of a mother's D-MER does not worsen in time. Once D-MER is part of the mother's lactation period, it will not increase in it's intensity presentation. Two things to be noted on this though; there

34

are things that can aggravate D-MER to make it temporarily feel worse, and the presentation of intensity can, and will, alleviate steadily over time.

What D-MER Feels Like For A Mother
Each mother's plight of D-MER will be unique to her. Her emotional radar, interpretation and past experiences will affect the way she interprets her emotions, as well as the spectrum and intensity of her D-MER. Again, D-MER has three different emotional spectrums that it can manifest in and the spectrum of a mother's D-MER will dictate how her D-MER feels. Below is a list of the most commonly used words that mothers use to explain her emotional reaction (see figures 1-3).

Despondent Spectrum
Angst
Apprehension
Blah feeling
Bothered
Concern
Depressed
Desire to be alone
Despair
Discouragement
Disheartened
Emotional upset
Exhaustion
Fatigued
Fear of having failed
General negative emotions
Gross

Guilt
Harmful thoughts
Hollow feeling in stomach
Homesickness
Hopelessness
Ickyness
Ill at Ease
Inability to cope
Introspective
Intrusive thoughts
Low mood
Low self-esteem
Oversensitivity
Sadness
Self Disgust
Sensation of a lump in the throat
Sensation of pit in stomach
Shame
Suicidal thoughts
Tearful
Unhappy
Urge to "get away"
Weepy
Worthlessness
Worrisome
Yuckyness

Anxiety Spectrum
Annoyance
Anxiety
Anxiousness
Dread

Frustration
Impatience
Irritability
Panic
Resentfulness
Restlessness

Agitation Spectrum
Aggressiveness
Agitation
Anger
Distress
Hostility
Paranoia
Tension

Mothers explain their feelings in different ways. Some examples of those portrayals are shared in these mother's testimonies:

It's like that flip flop of hollow panic in the center of your gut when your child falls off the monkey bars and you think it might be serious, or when you think an officer is going to pull you over but find out he's after someone else, or when you momentarily loose track of your child at the store.

It's like a horrible sadness in the center of your abdomen when you hurt your best friend's feelings and you think you may not be able to fix it, or when it's been a horrible day and you feel like you have no one to talk to, or when you feel like nothing you ever do turns out right and you might as well give up.

It's like a pit of guilt in your stomach, like when the cashier miscounts the change in your favor and you walk out of the store even though you knew of the error, or the feeling you get when everyone is so proud of what you did, but you know you cheated to get there.

It's like the feeling of the dread that you feel in your center when you have to take an exam you are not prepared for, or when you made a bad decision and cannot take it back.

It's like the churning angst you get in your middle when your name gets drug through the mud, or when someone you care about corrects you in front of important people and embarrasses you, or when you find out about horrible rumors that have been spread about you. It's how you feel when everybody is going to know it was you, what you said, or what you did, and how very wrong it was.

It's like the feeling of introspectiveness you get deep inside when there's no going back, when you cannot fix something unbearably wrong, when you feel completely off course. It's a feeling like.... life is very wrong and you do not know where to start.

For me it felt like a devil talked through my thoughts. I felt down, guilty and desperate. All very intensely.

We had a teacher at school who gave you his 'disappointed look' which was far worse than any other punishment. D-MER is like that feeling of having let everyone down and seeing no way out of the terrible thing you've done.

It's like everything in the room is suddenly happening very far off in the distance. It's a slow plummet to a disconnection from everyone around you. It's feeling incredibly homesick. It's floating above yourself and knowing that you can not float back down because your baby needs you. It's a craving for food or drink that does not exist. It's walking slowly into a deep pool, knowing that soon you will not be able to touch the bottom.

It feels like not feeling safe where you are and wanting to run away, but everywhere else seems even more scary. It's like homesickness even though you're sitting on the couch. It's like a moment of blind fear that you cannot talk yourself down from. It's wanting a hug from something that does not exist and even if it did you would not be able to find the words to ask.

It feels like every ounce of happiness is being pulled out of my body. I once heard someone describe it as the dementors from Harry Potter. I feel helpless, alone, like I could crawl in a hole and die. I feel like I want to crawl out of my own skin. It's an overwhelming feeling of dread.

It feels like the worst case of homesickness I ever felt and I had the most horrible feelings and thoughts within a split second. It made my eyes suddenly fill up with tears.

To me it feels like hopeless, like a ball of pain right in the center of the stomach that goes up to your chest and you freeze because you feel too scared to even move so you just hold the baby and wait until it passes but when it does you stay with a deep sadness and emptiness and a lump in your throat.

My heart skips a beat and I feel like I have to take a deep breath to get enough air and then I just want to cry, but I do not know why. It's like I get anxious and sad and I can not stop the feeling from coming.

I was feeling guilty for the feeling of D-MER, if that makes sense. At times I was also feeling angry, I hated myself as I thought there is something wrong with me and it's just me. I dreaded every feed.

It feels like you have made an unforgivable mistake. It feels as though you have killed someone and massive guilt and dread and shame are crushing you.

The best way I always described D-MER was that it felt like there was a dementor in the room. It did not necessarily turn cold, but it felt like all of your hope and happiness was being drained out of you.

To me, for about 30 seconds after every letdown, it felt like somebody had just told me the child in my arms had died.

Sudden and excessive unquenchable thirst and an overwhelming feeling of utter sadness and despair that rolls over me like a wave. Like the whole world rests on my shoulders and there is no hope. I breathe through it until it passes almost like through a contraction when in labour.

I described it as peeking through the keyhole of depression's door, without actually opening the door and walking in. A sense of helplessness and desperation for about 40 seconds to a minute or two and then, like nothing happened, back to normal.

It's that feeling when your boss calls and says, "Come down to my office, we need to talk about something" every time I had a letdown. The only way I got through it was by understanding the physiologic basis of it, anticipating the exact moment it would roll over me, and counting to ten waiting for it to end. Realizing it was a chemical reaction made it a million times easier to withstand it.

As if there is a horrible monster waiting in the pit of your stomach to pounce and when you do something as beautiful as feed your baby this dark feeling of dread washes over you, that nasty monster has pounced and cast dread and guilt and despair over you. Or you're doing something normal like washing up and the feeling comes over you and you feel so dark and sad that you could not even bring tears to your eyes all you can do is stare and stew on this sick sad feeling where you do not want to be alive.

My milk started coming in that very night. I guess with the pain that I still had with latching, I did not notice the D-MER the first few weeks. Soon though I began to worry about PPD. I would be in the shower and as spontaneous let downs happened over and over my skin crawled and I would sob with anger. I asked my husband if it seemed to him like I was off, but only when I nursed. I felt like there was a correlation, and so did he. I would close my eyes when I would nurse, instead of looking down at my sweet baby. I did not want her to see the sadness, anger, nausea, self disgust and confusion that crossed over my eyes while my milk let down to feed my daughter. I would tell her, "It's not you baby girl, it's not you". My sweet toddler wanted to come see the baby feeding, and I would have to say, "please, just wait". I felt like it took all my energy to even get those words out. I would feel my whole body either sink into what felt like a never ending hole. My toes would curl as my body recoiled from this terrifying feeling. I have talked to everyone I know about it. Some people believe me, some people do not. But along the way I have met many who did not even know it was a real thing. Some even family members. I am 4 months postpartum, it's not always as bad, it goes in waves, but it's not gone. Like a nightmare inside my body stealing what could be beautiful.

Dementors

D-MER is so frequently likened to how Dementors are represented in the popular literary series of Harry Potter, that it is uncanny. In her blog, "Mummy's Little Monkey", a mother with D-MER shared, *"it (letdown) was like the Dementors were nearby, and were sucking all the light and joy out of the room."* Mothers make this parallel based on the author J.K. Rowling's descriptions in her book as well as from the depictions of the Dementor's affects on people from the films, that are based on the books. Here is one YouTube link of Dementors in action. Dementors are mainly relatable to mothers with D-MER for two reasons; one is because their power and purpose is to literally emotionally soul suck it's victim and two, because the effect they have happens very fast; though if they are fought off, the victim quickly recovers

42

emotionally and is back to normal. Much like a D-MER episode. One mother wrote in her blog "Natalie's Sentiments", *"It was as if all the color in the world drained and I would never feel happiness again. Every negative emotion converged at once. I remember seeing the Dementors in Harry Potter and yelling "that's what it feels like when I nurse!"* If someone is already familiar with the fictional demon, than this analogy can easily make sense. For others that may not have a frame of reference for Dementors, a young author depicts Rowling's creatures as follows.

"Dementors are among the foulest creatures that walk this earth. They infest the darkest, filthiest places, they glory in decay and despair, they drain peace, hope, and happiness out of the air around them. ... Get too near a Dementor and every good feeling, every happy memory will be sucked out of you."

These words are from Harry Potter and the Prisoner of Azkaban by J.K. Rowling. With them, she describes dementors, creatures that feed on human souls.

Dementors (their name, a blend of 'torment' and 'dement') are hooded, wraith-like creatures whose forms resemble those of humans, but have the appearance of a grey, decaying body. They consume the souls of humans, but in doing so, they quite literally suck the happiness out of their victims and thus leave those anywhere near them with feelings of utter depression and despair. Upon eating a soul, a dementor leaves their victims like an empty shell; a functioning being with a heart that pumps and lungs that breath, but with nothing else.

It is widely known that these creatures and the effects they have on humans were based on the feelings that Rowling experienced during her battle with depression[1], and it's an incredibly accurate interpretation.

Being so directly linked to depression, it is also a widely chosen comparison to the feeling of d-mer. However, one is not left defenseless to the power of dementors. It is possible to cast a Patronus charm, described in the book as 'a kind of Anti-Dementor – a guardian which acts as a shield between you and the Dementor.' It's also 'a kind of positive force, a projection of the very things that the Dementor feeds upon – hope, happiness, the desire to survive – but it cannot feel despair, as real humans can, so the Dementors can't hurt it.' So while darkness and the consumption of souls exists, so does light and the protection of souls.

It is my personal hope, and the hope of many, that d-mer mothers will be able to find their patronuses through further world-wide education and research concerning dysphoric milk ejection reflex. While it may seem bleak, we have only to continue to learn so that we might protect and defend ourselves and fight for our souls and our well being.

Written by Faeli (Felicia) Heise

How D-MER Affects A Mother
D-MER can cause a cascade of challenges and negative circumstances. It can cause a mother to doubt her own

---

[1] Depression and Dementors: the magic of Harry Potter and grief by Lauren Entwistle

emotional experience and the validity of her emotions, it can affect the family as the mother struggles to get through her D-MER episodes, it puts the mother at risk for early weaning, it takes a higher than average mental and emotional toll on the breastfeeding mother, and it can cause a new mother who already feels a new kind of social isolation, to feel even more isolated because of the lack of awareness and understanding of her situation.

Marcelina Watkinson, DClinPsy, who did research about the difference between breastfeed aversion and D-MER found that mothers who already had a vulnerability to depression and self-harm, were taken back to those experiences when experiencing D-MER.[2] She also says, "the other thing 'my' mothers reported was how the experiences interfered with their identity as a "good mother", because the D-MER experiences during breastfeeding were in such stark contrast to what they had anticipated what breastfeeding would be like and the closeness with the baby that it was going to result in."

A mother with D-MER is going through many devastating emotional episodes each day, with each feeding and with each spontaneous letdown, only to return to feeling like her normal self within a few minutes, and she can be greatly affected by this. This is especially true for mothers who do

---

[2] Maternal experiences of embodied emotional sensations during breast feeding: An Interpretative Phenomenological Analysis: Marcelina Watkinson, DClinPsy (Dr), Craig Murray, PhD, DHealthPsy (Dr), Jane Simpson, PhD, DClinPsy (Dr) Division of Health Research, Furness College, Lancaster University, Lancaster LA1 4YG, United Kingdom

not know what is happening to them or why, as well as for mothers who have more severe cases that have the most intense negative emotional reactions with D-MER. The confusion as well as the exhaustion of the D-MER episodes can be very taxing.

Often mothers feel alone and isolated in their challenge and can feel disconnected from support, information or peers. Mothers are usually quite uncertain and hesitate about speaking up about what they are feeling. They have later reported that they stayed quiet about what they were going through because they felt "like a freak", like a "bad mother" and "weird" for their emotional reaction. In societies where women already struggle with the validation of their emotions, it is hardly surprising that there is hesitancy about speaking about negative emotions during breastfeeding inside a lactation community, to a partner, or in any mother-to-mother sharing.

It can be hard for a mother to articulate her feelings to another and to feel understood by others about the struggle within her experience. It is not only a very odd emotional trial, but it is one that can be predicted and measured. It is one that can cause feelings that range from wistful to angry, depending on the mother's spectrum, and it is over before she can even begin to evaluate what she is feeling, or why.

It may cause mothers to over think and over evaluate their life and themselves. This is understandable because it is normal and reasonable, that when someone experiences an emotion, that they connect it to an event or experience. This leads a woman to spend a lot of mental energy trying to figure out what happened in her last hour, day, or life that has caused her to feel so many negative emotions. In the case of D-MER though, there is no rational or logical connection to truly be made. The emotional reaction happens because of the milk ejection being triggered, and not because of anything in the woman's day. When a mother does not understand what is happening to her, there is no way to gain perspective on this though, and a mother who is educated about her D-MER, still spends precious energy reminding herself that she does not need to address or fix her emotional state, as it is not a reaction to an event.

D-MER can cause mothers to dread breastfeeding. Considering that breastfeeding is often viewed as a positive experience, a chance to slow down, and an opportunity to bond with the baby, it can be very discouraging to a mother for this opportunity to be turned into something negative. For most breastfeeding mothers in established lactation, the opportunity to sit down and feed the baby can be a welcome break, or it can be something she can do without even hardly thinking about it, often carrying on other tasks while she feeds her baby. This is not the case for a mother with D-MER. There may be apprehension and dread associated with feedings, the feeds take her out of the moment and they demand her attention and derail her daily flow. This can be intrusive and depleting to a mother.

Often mothers need to distract themselves from their emotions while feeding, and will utilize the TV, her phone, a book or another tool. This can be a helpful way of coping, but it is unfortunate in itself because these methods also distract her from things she would otherwise be desiring to pay attention to, such as a partner, a task at hand, her other children, or her nursing baby. Other mothers find that mindfulness and acceptance of her experience can make it more manageable, using meditation, deep breathing or other mindfulness techniques. This can ease the mother's emotional toll from D-MER but it, too, takes an emotional and mental focus away from other things.

As if these things collectively were not of concern, all of these points can of course also put the mother at a greater chance for weaning sooner than she or her baby would prefer.

Self Directed Feelings

It is common for people to wonder where a mother with D-MER projects her feelings. It is true that D-MER happens for physiological reasons but because of its emotionally based reaction, it begs the question as to what the mother's emotional response to the reaction is. Many have made the assumption that a mother blames the baby or holds resentment that the baby is responsible for her feelings, but this has not shown to be the case at all. It is known that the feelings of D-MER are, in most cases, not directed towards the baby and that they manifest completely separately from the child. The feelings tend to be self-directed and projected onto the mother's own immediate world and experiences, aside from her infant. There are not thoughts towards the baby about the baby being responsible for the emotional state, mothers do not report frustration or anger towards the baby, and mothers do not blame or resent the baby for their feelings. A mother is more likely to think *"what is wrong with me?"* over *"why are you doing this to me?"* Instead, the mother seems to take a self-directed approach to the interpretation to her feelings. In this way she may feel like something is wrong with her, she is bad, she is failing, she is to blame, or that she has done something wrong (see figure 19). At times mothers have talked about being so overwhelmed with their emotional reaction that their outward response may be projected externally, with a sharp word to her partner, impatience shown to an older child, or impatience with someone else around her. But when this does happen, mothers have never reported holding other people responsible for the feelings that are manifesting inside of her. Mothers either hold themselves, or D-MER responsible for the feelings. The outward portrayal of emotion appears to happen more often with mothers with agitation D-MER, less so with anxiety D-MER and rarely with despondency D-MER. A mother with anxiety D-MER divulged, *"I'm not even 2 weeks into breastfeeding my second child, I've had D-MER both times. I feel like I get anxious leading up to a feed, and then when the D-MER hits I get all these horrible thoughts and feelings, and then after the feed I feel guilty and I get cranky and take it out on my toddler and partner."* It is more likely for mothers with anxiety and agitation D-MER to have more outward expressions and responses most likely because agitation and anger is naturally an emotion that pulls for an external response towards others, in contrast to sadness or depression which many find to be more of a private or internal experience.

Feeling Like A Bad Mother
It is not uncommon for the self directed feelings of D-MER to result in the direct projection of feeling like a bad mother

49

in general. A mother admitted, "at *first I felt like a horrible mother for feeling that way about breastfeeding my son whom I love so much. I felt like a monster!*" It is not surprising that mothers struggle with their sense of worth when dealing with D-MER. New mothers often struggle with their worthiness as they settle into mothering a new child and mother with D-MER may noticed a weighted challenge in this. D-MER can easily portray itself as emotions of self disgust, self doubt, shame and guilt. Breastfeeding itself is generally held in lofty adoration as a wonderful, warm and fuzzy bonding experience, but if a mother is having adverse emotions when breastfeeding, including ones of self disgust or shame, the self directed projection of feeling like she is a failure as a mother is not a far reach for her to make. A mother with D-MER benefits from support and education because then she can consciously release herself from her blame and self accusation.

Intrusive Thoughts

The negative emotional experience is likely to be followed by unsettling or unpleasant thoughts. This is basic biology. Negative emotional encounters have the power to alter the way we see ourselves, others, and the world. With a mother with D-MER, what was good and okay only moments ago, can quickly feel bad and become distorted upon letdown. She may simply be trying to decide what to make her family for dinner when her dysphoria hits her, and she could easily project her physiological reaction into a psychological conclusion, perhaps chastising herself for not having enough healthy food options in the home for her family or some other valid, but seemingly irrational verdict. This is one of the main reasons why it is so important for a mother to understand that her emotional interlude is beyond her control. With so many seemingly random negative emotional reactions every day, it can become all too easy for a mother to start second guessing herself, her choices and her life. There can become a near constant rollercoaster of viewing her circumstances as normal and good before crashing down into a place where she cannot figure out where she went wrong. In severe cases it is not unheard of for these self doubts to turn into self criticism in a way that can truly concern a mother. Thoughts of self-harm and suicidal ideation can be part of D-MER. This is not uncommon and though it is scary, it is assuredly not rare with D-MER. There have been only two reports, however, of mothers acting in a self harming manner during a D-MER episode. Generally it seems that mothers are able to move through the intrusive thoughts without feeling compelled to act on them. This is more easily done when the mother understands that her emotions are caused by the MER and not because of valid emotional self loathing. It stands to reiterate, that D-MER is generally not an emotional event that is projected onto the nursing infant, the intrusive thoughts are not about the baby, and that D-MER is a very self directed happening. Mothers who do have thoughts of self harm, who are concerned about acting on these thoughts and urges, are directed to bring this to the attention of a medical professional immediately. Mothers who do not fit the trend of self-directed thoughts and feelings and are concerned about the thoughts and feelings that they have towards their baby or towards others are also advised to seek help and support immediately. Severe cases of D-MER and mothers who have extenuating circumstances or uncharacteristic D-MER need additional help and support with their situation.

Cognitive Distortions

A mother with D-MER can be affected by poor and negative cognitive functions that can manifest from her dysphoria. Cognitive distortions (such as all or nothing thinking, projection, personalization, and others) can be a struggle to avoid for a mother who has a hard time separating herself from her emotions during the milk release. Some mothers with D-MER, once learning of it's physiological foundation, can easily separate themselves from the negative feelings and they do not cause them much further cognitive distress. Other mothers find that it is much harder for them to separate themselves from it, and the more severe the D-MER is, the harder it is for a mother to manage. When a mother cannot mentally and emotionally divorce herself from her dysphoria then she is likely to unconsciously pursue varies cognitive distortions in her mind. Cognitive distortions are inaccurate thoughts that the mind uses to convince oneself of something that is not true about an emotional experience. For example, someone may cheat, then feel guilty, and in response blame someone else. The blame (a cognitive distortion) is used to help the person avoid the uncomfortable feeling of guilt. For a mother with D-MER there is no justifiable cause for her emotions (she did not cheat), but she may feel guilty during D-MER, and in response she may find herself dealing with it through the use of cognitive distortions. Cognitive distortions are considered rather ineffective coping tools to help the brain handle emotions. Some of them are more mature than others, for example intellectualization. Some are more immature, such as projection. For a mother to separate herself from her feelings by understanding D-MER is the antagonist of them, she is ultimately intellectualizing her experience and this can be a healthy way for her to manage her D-MER. Some mothers may struggle to do this for various reasons and a mother may find herself projecting her feelings of guilt (or otherwise) onto something else, like the credit card balance that she has been neglecting. The kind of interpersonal awareness it takes to choose more advanced cognitive coping mechanisms is a skill that can be learned and it can aid a mother in managing her feelings more easily.

Familiar Feelings Of D-MER

Some mothers, though by no means all, report that the brief feeling of D-MER is a sensation that feels familiar to them from other times in their life. One mother wrote, *"for me, it's sheer panic, a moment where I lose my breath and my heart beats rapidly, and then a feeling of heartache, longing, or homesickness. Sometimes I equate it to the feeling I had as a kid, being scared to go in the basement alone. I would run up the stairs as fast as I could, petrified that someone was going to grab me from behind. So weird that this happens during breastfeeding."* Of course in all ways emotions all familiar, it is learned at a young age how to put names to feelings and mothers with D-MER have no problem doing the same; picking out words like dread or sadness or anxiety. But there seems to sometimes be something more distinctive for mothers as they feel their D-MER; they can also feel like it is a familiar recognition. It can feel like a ghost-like dysphoria that is somehow linked to something unique that they have felt before, but a feeling that they can not quite place, remember or explain in detail. One mother shared, *"it was the same feeling I had sometimes as a child, it is similar to the feeling of being homesick/bad feeling in the stomach.*

I could get the feeling out of nothing as a child, and it would go away as quickly as it came. Even when I was home and doing nothing." Another mother put into words, *"it felt like homesickness. The same feeling I would get as a kid when I would sleep over at a friend's house, just 100 times worse."* It is true that many mothers remember vague childhood feelings of distress, loneliness, homesickness or unhappiness that suddenly reappear in the form of D-MER. But not all mothers connect it to unplaceable childhood sensations. One mother expressed it as, *"I can liken it to is when people say somebody has stepped on your grave".* This is a very distinct déjà vu kind of description; something vague, unsettling and familiar. This correlation does not indicate childhood trauma, repressed memories or a history of abuse, by any means. Not all mothers with D-MER feel this kind of ghost type dysphoria with D-MER, and the more likely explanation is just the history and repetition of the hormonal cocktail that happens with D-MER. As another mother communicated, *"D-MER reflected feelings I experienced as a kid, maybe I was feeling isolated, or socially anxious, or really insecure about an idea or expression. D-MER felt almost nostalgic to me. I think for whatever reason my brain has created a pathway towards shame after joy is experienced. This could have been conditioned subtly. Or not so subtly if in the case of abuse. Creating new pathways in the brain is used in all sorts of rehabilitations and I think it's possible for the D-MER to be "rewired". The amount of women who recognize the commonalities of D-MER to these other dysphoric experiences is so overwhelming that the connection cannot be ignored."*

Disgust Reaction

Mothers with D-MER often use the word disgust. This is how experiencing nausea with milk release can be misconstrued as D-MER, because some mothers do feel nausea with letdown. But for mothers who feel only nausea with letdown, it is an isolated physical reaction to milk release, with no emotional component. Alternatively, mothers with D-MER experience a disgust reaction as part of their dysphoria, easily labeled as nausea. Dopamine suppression suppresses appetitive seeking [3], and sometimes food intake as well.[4] This is why mothers can report feeling hungry before a D-MER episode, and can immediately push away a plate of food when the dysphoria hits, often regaining her appetite as soon as her letdowns are complete. As one mother related, *"the worst is when D-MER comes right when your food is set down in front of you! I completely lose my appetite even if I was starving to begin with. I regain my appetite soon after the D-MER ends"*. It appears that often the disgust reaction with D-MER is both a physical and emotional sensation, the physical part being that of the stomach turning in disgust while the mother in turn feels emotionally disgusted. A mother articulated, *"I have been nursing my son for four months now and although I do not feel it every time, and*

[3] Behav Pharmacol. 2013 Dec; 24(8): 633–639. The dopamine D2 antagonist eticlopride accelerates extinction and delays reacquisition of food self-administration in rats
Jonathon Koerber, David Goodman, Jesse L. Barnes, and Jeffrey W. Grimm

[4] Front Neuroendocrinol. 2010 Jan;31(1):104-12. doi: 10.1016/j.yfrne.2009.10.004. Epub 2009 Oct 28.
Metabolic hormones, dopamine circuits, and feeding. Narayanan NS1, Guarnieri DJ, DiLeone RJ.

sometimes it's fleeting, I still get it. I feel this awful sad/ disgusting/immoral feeling in the pit of my stomach, and it makes me feel like I'm terrible." The feeling of disgust with D-MER seems to be multifaceted.

Misinterpretation Of D-MER

It is not uncommon for mothers to be confused or baffled by their experience and can often confuse D-MER for something else. Fortunately as awareness is spread and information about D-MER becomes more readily available online, this becomes less common. But there are some factors that can cause mothers, or health care professionals, to misinterpret a mother's concerns.

Sometimes a mother does not feel a physical letdown sensation in her breasts. This can make it harder for her to connect her emotional feelings to her milk letdown. When a mother has the physical cue of a tingling in her breasts right after her initial emotional drop, she can more quickly connect the phenomenon of one to the other. If she does not have the physical cue, the emotional drop can seem much more random and unexplainable.

For the same reason, if there is no leaking with a spontaneous letdown of milk, then a mother may not have as much of a tangible connection of emotional low and milk ejection reflex. Spontaneous letdowns are something that happen when a mother is not nursing. The occurrence of spontaneous letdown seems to be a very common reason for mothers to misinterpret their experience and cause them to take longer to connect their abrupt dysphoria to the MER.

Spontaneous letdowns happen for a variety of reasons outside the nipple stimulation of a pump or baby. Spontaneous letdowns can be caused by anything from over fullness of the breasts, a crying baby, thinking about nursing, or sexual arousal. A mother may be aware of these letdowns, which is in her favor because she will be more likely to connect her dysphoria to the MER. But if a mother does not have physical letdown sensations or leaking, then she has no way of knowing that her dysphoria is connected to milk release. This means that she could readily connect dysphoria to nursing when she is actively nursing, but then dismiss the connection when she knows that the emotional drop happens at other times when she is not nursing. This could keep a mother from being able to ask the right questions or find the right help for her concerns.

Another factor that can cause D-MER to be unrecognized for what it is, is the fact that there are multiple letdowns per feeding.[5] Since there are many letdowns per feeding, there may not be the tell tale strong and distinctive emotional dips and surges. A mother with D-MER may have barely recovered from her first dysphoric drop of the first letdown, when her baby has already stimulated another release causing dopamine to once again act inappropriately. This would cause a mother to stay in a near constant state of dysphoria until her MERs space themselves out, slow down, stop or the baby ends the feeding. Since D-MER is generally described as a repetitive experience that lasts about 2

[5] Pediatrics February 2004, VOLUME 113 / ISSUE 2 Ultrasound Imaging of Milk Ejection in the Breast of Lactating Women Donna T. Ramsay, Jacqueline C. Kent, Robyn A. Owens, Peter E. Hartmann

minutes, a mother who feels like her dysphoria lasts 10-15 minutes may think that she is struggling with something different. It is most common for mothers to notice the dips and surges of dysphoria, usually the first one being the most intense. But there are times that mothers have had letdowns so close together during feedings that there is very little relief and the wave like sensation is less pronounced.

A major factor in not recognizing D-MER for what it is, is the incredible amount of awareness that has been spread about postpartum depression. If a new mother has complaints of a low mood they are almost always immediately associated with PPD. Mothers with D-MER may initially think and ask about "PPD that happens now and again" or "PPD that comes and goes". These are common phrases that can be clues that D-MER is present. But if a mother or healthcare professional is unaware of D-MER, than it can quickly and easily be misdiagnosed as postpartum depression. This can lead to a mother being treated with medications that are unnecessary and will not help her D-MER. The majority of medications that are prescribed for PPD are serotonin reuptake inhibitors (SSRI's) and D-MER's seemingly malfunctioning neurotransmitter is dopamine.

Last but not least, a major reason for the misunderstanding of a mother's experience is the lack of knowledge about D-MER. It is very hard to recognize and accept something that is not known about or understood. But just as PPD used to be unrecognized and misunderstood, and is now given the awareness and attention that is needed, the hope is that D-MER is not far behind in also being more widely known.

Chapter Three
What Has Been Concluded About D-MER

It stands to say again, that from an evidence based perspective, less is known about D-MER than is known; the evidence base is limited. Many mothers, however, initially care less about evidence based information, than they do about knowing that they are not alone. So first and foremost it is important to state that it is known that a negative emotional reaction to the milk ejection reflex is something that a lactating mother may experience. It is something that happens, so yes, it is real. This reaction to milk letdown has come to be known by way of reference, as dysphoric milk ejection reflex. With that basic information in hand, and without D-MER being studied beyond case reports, anecdotal reports and limited qualitatative research, it makes it difficult to make robust scientific statements about D-MER. However, science is continuously evolving, which broadens the foundation for new concepts to be known and understood. As D-MER becomes more studied, some of what seems to be known now, may be overwritten. In the meantime, however, some initial conclusions can be put forth.

The Involvement Of Dopamine
Following preliminary exploration of the links between D-MER and maternal coping mechanisms, it has been speculated that dopamine may play an important role in the experience of D-MER. In the first case study of D-MER, it emerged that certain substances, such as nicotine, large amounts of chocolate ice cream and pseudoephedrine (taken

to alleviate a cold) also seemed to alleviate D-MER, or temporarily improve it.[6] However, many of them were not safe or sustainable options for the ongoing correction of D-MER, and are therefore not recommended. However, it was observed that all of these interventions did ease the mother's D-MER for brief amounts of time, and as referenced in the original case report, these particular substances elevate dopamine levels temporarily. The corollary of this is that gently supporting dopamine levels in a mother with D-MER may ease her dysphoria. D-MER at a glance is not a mood disorder. Mothers with D-MER often feel normal and stable aside from their dysphoric episodes, so unlike other mood disorders that require constant regulation of the neurotransmitters, D-MER may only need minimal intervention. There is no drug designed for this purpose, but as mothers have shared and reported on their individual efforts to alleviate their D-MER, it has been observed that some natural approaches to supporting a mother's dopamine levels have had positive effects on D-MER. Furthermore, a few anecdotal reports from mothers with D-MER suggest that safely, slightly and gently supporting dopamine levels with medication seems to alleviate the negative emotional reaction to the milk ejection reflex. In summary, mothers have found some relief by trying a few particular herbs, medications and vitamins that support the availability of dopamine in the body and there have been some initial encouraging success stories with some of these treatments. It is this pattern that points towards dopamine possibly being

---

[6] Heise AM, Wiessinger D. Dysphoric milk ejection reflex: A case report. Int Breastfeed J. 2011 Jun 6;6(1):6.

involved in the experience of D-MER. The supposed mechanism is explained further in following chapters.

How Education Helps

All mothers with D-MER find great relief and comfort in being educated about what may be the cause of their problem, finding peer support and being validated by others when sharing their experience and struggles. Many do not seek any correction or intervention beyond that. D-MER primarily affects how a mother may think about herself or her current experience. For example, *"I feel sad so therefore something must be wrong"*. However, frequently mothers discover that this is often not the case. Mothers often find great solace in the fact that though her body may be betraying her by sending inappropriate signals to her brain, her life is indeed not falling apart and is not in need of constant reevaluation. One mother stated, *"the one thing that helped was to know that I was not crazy for feeling that way and that there were many other women struggling with the same condition. Also knowing that it was not going to be permanent."* It is normal for someone to want to have an understanding of their emotionally upsetting episodes. For a mother with D-MER it becomes clearer to her that the intense emotional disruption is directly linked to a physiological response. This is a rare combination and its particular, distinct, consistent and repetitive action is unlike anything else currently known of. The experience may cause a mother significant confusion and distress, resulting in a mistrust in herself and her interpretations. Simple education about D-MER goes an incredible length in settling and encouraging a mother with D-MER.

Difference From Other Uncomfortable Feelings

There are, indeed, a variety of situations that can cause mothers to feel uncomfortable with or when breastfeeding. However, D-MER has its own markers and distinctions that set it apart from other breastfeeding discomforts. D-MER is not a general dislike of breastfeeding, impatience with baby at the breast, irritability from nipple pain, breastfeeding aversion, postpartum depression, suppressed trauma, or sadness during pumping because of separation from the baby. All of these things can certainly be triggers of strong distressing emotional reactions during breastfeeding, but they do not bear the consistent markers of distinction that D-MER has. In the majority of cases when a breastfeeding mother with D-MER comes across this knowledge, she immediately resonates with the information and recognizes that D-MER is indeed what she is being affected by. Often if a mother is being affected by some other emotional or mood related experience when breastfeeding, the information on D-MER may somewhat resonate but will often still leave her doubtful about this explanation of her experiences. D-MER tends to be highly reliable, distinct and definitive in its presentation.

Reoccurrence Of D-MER

The trend, so often reported with mothers with D-MER, is that once a mother experiences it with one child, she will have the same experience with future children. Rarely does it happen that a mother does not continue to experience D-MER with subsequent children. However, it is completely possible that a mother will not have D-MER with her first or second child, but once the hormonal activity around the MER changes, D-MER is continued in future lactations.

Stories of the mothers that have shared their experiences suggest that reoccurrence of D-MER is nearly always guaranteed.

When D-MER Starts To Manifest

D-MER seems to most commonly start to manifest upon the occurrence of lactogenesis II, which is the onset of copious milk secretion occurring between 32-96 hours postpartum.[7] This is known as the mother's milk "coming in". Some mothers may not notice D-MER this early, with many other emotions and challenges in front of her. This is especially true if her D-MER is more of a mild manifestation. Many mothers have reported starting to notice the surges and relief pattern of negative emotions, and subsequently connecting them to letdown by 2-4 weeks postpartum. If a mother feels that her D-MER started later than 1-2 months into lactation, it would be well worth it to look closer and make sure that it is not another concern or issue that is similar to D-MER, as it does not seem to be typical for D-MER to manifest so late into established lactation. General depression or anxiety, a change in the mother's life, panic disorder, breastfeeding aversion, the start of a new medication or galactagogue or other medical issues should be investigated as well, if a mother is complaining of negative feelings in a later stage of lactation.

---

[7] 2001 The American Society for Nutritional Sciences Physiology and Endocrine Changes Underlying Human Lactogenesis II1,2 Margaret C. Neville*,3 and Jane Morton†

Duration Of D-MER During Lactation

The length and longevity of D-MER appears to be determined by the severity of the experience. The more severe a mother's D-MER, the longer the D-MER is likely to last through her breastfeeding journey. For mothers with a milder experience, the D-MER may self-correct within 3-6 months. Mothers that have severe instances find that even if their baby nurses into toddlerhood, that the D-MER may persevere throughout. Regardless, it is often the case that the further into the breastfeeding journey, the easier D-MER becomes. This is not only because a mother often finds support and tools to make the trial less uncomfortable, but also because the distressing hormonal reaction to the MER seems to ease as the baby gets older. Logically this could be because as milk regulation becomes more stable, as the baby becomes more efficient at the breast and, in time, as the milk volume decreases as the baby takes nutrients from other sources; the prolactin levels are likely to change. In response, the correlation and relationship that prolactin has to dopamine may alter in such a way that the dysphoria is not as prevalent. Regardless of what the scientific explanation may be for the eventual self-correction of D-MER, it seems to happen between 3 months and 2 years the majority of the time.

Physical Experience Of D-MER

Many people ask if there are physical symptoms that are connected to D-MER. In short, no, not directly. D-MER has an emotional component, above all else. There are some breastfeeding women who experience physical anomalies when letting down their milk. Some complain of headaches, or break out in hives, experience nausea, or have an uncomfortable sensation in their breasts. These, and other isolated physical symptoms, are not associated with D-MER. It is not uncommon, however, for mothers with D-MER to report some physical changes when they experience D-MER. This should come as no surprise, however, as D-MER is an intense emotional and hormonal experience. Just as intense anxiety, anger or depression are emotional experiences that have bodily effects, so can D-MER. Some mothers may tear up, or feel a pit in their stomach (that can be interpreted as nausea), have an elevated heart rate, or feel generally physically unsettled. But it is important to note that these are most likely a result of her emotional response. Physical reactions to letdown are not currently in the criteria for determining if a mother has D-MER. If a mother does not have the tell-tale sign of a negative emotional and dysphoric emotional response with letdown, it is most likely not D-MER.

Difference From Breastfeeding Aversion

D-MER is different from what is known as nursing aversion.[8] Breastfeeding aversion can happen to some mothers when nursing while pregnant or nursing older toddlers. This happens upon nipple contact and does not have anything to do with the MER, but instead with the tactical sensation on

---

[8] Midwifery May 2016Volume 36, Pages 53–60 Maternal experiences of embodied emotional sensations during breast feeding: An Interpretative Phenomenological Analysis Marcelina Watkinson, DClinPsy (Dr) DClinPsy Marcelina Watkinson DClinPsy Marcelina Watkinson, Craig Murray, PhD, DHealthPsy (Dr) PhD, DHealthPsy Craig Murray, Jane Simpson, PhD, DClinPsy (Dr) PhD, DClinPsy Jane Simpson Division of Health Research, Furness College, Lancaster University, Lancaster LA1 4YG, United Kingdom

the nipple itself. D-MER starts within the first few weeks of the postpartum period, whereas breastfeeding aversion starts in late infancy or toddler hood and is often described as a body's biological way of moving the breastfeeding dyad towards natural weaning.[9] There have been mothers with D-MER that have nursed long enough to also experience nursing aversion and the explanations of the difference in sensation and emotion are quite stark differences. Breastfeeding aversion is by far the most common experience misinterpreted as D-MER, by mothers, that has been noticed thus far. More can be learned about breastfeeding aversion in the book, Adventures in Tandem Nursing by Hilary Flower.

Difference From Postpartum Depression
D-MER is seemingly not associated with postpartum depression and it is not currently recognized as a kind of type of postpartum depression or a postpartum mood disorder. Some of the differences between postpartum depression and D-MER include that D-MER comes and goes in waves, unlike PPD which is a steady and consistent mood disorder. It has also been shown that the medications most often used to treat PPD in lactating women (usually sertraline, also known as Zoloft) have no effect on D-MER. Most medications that treat PPD are serotonin reuptake inhibitors, which work by blocking the reabsorption (reuptake) of serotonin in the brain, making more serotonin available. Since D-MER is likely to be dopamine mediated, this class of drugs is seemingly ineffective on D-MER. A

---

[9] Breastfeeding Agitation Hilary Flower St. Petersburg FL USA LEAVEN, Vol. 39 No. 4, August-September 2003, pp. 90-91.

mother with D-MER may have PPD as well as D-MER and PPD could be exacerbated by the experience of D-MER as it further reinforces to the mother her existing experience of all those distressing feelings. Otherwise, D-MER and PPD are separate and unrelated. The misdiagnosis by doctors of D-MER as postpartum depression is the most common misdiagnosis reported thus far.[10]

Physiological Reaction With A Psychological Response

D-MER is triggered by a physiological reaction and not a psychological one. It is true, however, that a psychological reaction is often triggered. Indeed, all emotional reactions have accompanied physiological and cognitive responses. However, while a mother with post traumatic stress disorder (PTSD) from sexual assault may have an anxious response to nipple stimulation from the baby, or a mother with postpartum depression may feel additional sadness when trying to bond with her baby through breastfeeding; a mother with D-MER experiences dysphoria when the milk ejection reflex is triggered. This is a psychological response to a physiological experience. For a mother grappling with the confusion of her roller coaster of unprecedented feelings, this is by far the simplest and most helpful explanation. It

---

[10] Midwifery May 2016Volume 36, Pages 53–60 Maternal experiences of embodied emotional sensations during breast feeding: An Interpretative Phenomenological Analysis Marcelina Watkinson, DClinPsy (Dr) DClinPsy Marcelina Watkinson DClinPsy Marcelina Watkinson, Craig Murray, PhD, DHealthPsy (Dr) PhD, DHealthPsy Craig Murray, Jane Simpson, PhD, DClinPsy (Dr) PhD, DClinPsy Jane Simpson Division of Health Research, Furness College, Lancaster University, Lancaster LA1 4YG, United Kingdom

seems that those with consistent mood disorders have an easier time understanding that they are having a psychological response to physiological issues. Additionally, many mood disorders do have life circumstance triggers and aggravators. Mothers with D-MER do not have the same consistent experience of some mood disorders. D-MER is not currently classified as a mood disorder, but it can be helpful to remember the cause and effect of physiological reactions with psychological responses in the body.

Chapter Four
What Is Being Deduced About D-MER

There are different ways to define what is "known" about D-MER, and this is heavily dependent on one's role in the lactation community. For mothers with D-MER, simply knowing that they are not alone can be enough. On the contrary, the medical and scientific community states that nothing is truly "known" about D-MER. It has been determined that there is a subset of mothers who have a negative emotional experience upon milk release that is surprisingly predictable and very similar to one another's. Aside from this, there is not much that we can say is strictly scientifically "known". However, regardless of what may actually be happening in the body and the brain, the effects and trends seem to follow undeniable patterns from which preliminary conclusions can be drawn, in order to try and support women.

The Mechanism Of D-MER

Lactation, though around since the dawn of mammals, is a new area of study. The true medical and scientific investigation of lactation has only been around since the 18th century, when the first medical comparison of human milk and other mammalian milk was done in 1790.[11] Early conclusions about lactation and its processes were based on information gathered using limited technology. It was not until the 1970's that the lactation process became better understood and breastfeeding rates began to rise again. It is proper and expected that there is still more to learn, find and understand.

The possible mechanism underlying D-MER has been inferred from what is currently known about lactation. The lactating woman is under the influence of many hormones and chemical processes. However, in the past years there have been two hormones that have been the main focus within lactation research; prolactin and oxytocin. These two hormones have two simple and unique jobs. Prolactin aids in the message sent to the body to make milk, and oxytocin is in charge of communicating that milk needs to be moved (causing the letdown reflex). Thus, as D-MER started to become an area of scientific inquiry, it was natural to look towards these hormones first. The neuropeptide oxytocin, is the hormone most highly associated with the MER. Oxytocin, however, is famous for its soothing, calming and

---

[11] J Perinat Educ. 2009 Spring; 18(2): 32–39. A History of Infant Feeding Emily E Stevens, RN, FNP, WHNP, PhD, Thelma E Patrick, RN, PhD, and Rita Pickler, RN, PNP, PhD

bonding effect. Not only in lactation, but in any experience in which oxytocin levels surge. With the knowledge that human emotional reactions result from the various neurotransmitter and hormonal activities in the brain, it was important to understand better what other brain functions play a part in lactation. Not surprisingly, it was discovered that in addition to prolactin and oxytocin, a number of other hormones and neurotransmitters are involved. Vasopressin and dopamine are also other two main players in the neurotransmitter and hormonal cocktail of lactation. However, for the purpose of understanding D-MER, the exploration of the role of dopamine is the focus. Dopamine is known as prolactin's "gatekeeper" or more technically, it is know as a prolactin inhibiting factor.[12] In order for prolactin levels to rise, dopamine has to get out of its way, and open the gate for it to rise (see figure 13). When the milk release is triggered in a mother, by nipple stimulation, over fullness of the breasts, or thoughts of the baby, oxytocin spikes and it does so quite quickly. This is to push the milk in the direction of the nipple. But at the same time, prolactin is triggered to start its slower rise, which prepares the body to make more milk for future feedings. Before prolactin can start this, however, dopamine must adjust itself slightly and drop its own levels to make way for prolactin. This all happens in every breastfeeding mother without her knowing it, and sometimes the only sign that it's happened is the tingling sensation in the breasts that can come once the milk starts moving, or she may know she's had a MER because of milk leaking or the baby's gulping.

---

[12] Behavioral Neuroendocrinology Page 253 Barry R. Komisaruk, Gabriela González-Mariscal - 2017

In a mother with D-MER it is believed that there is a slight variation of the process involving dopamine in the MER (see figure 14). For a mother who has dysphoria with MER, the process is more like this; the MER is triggered by one of the same stimuli, and oxytocin rises, prolactin communicates that it is time to rise and thusly, dopamine drops, but in the situation of D-MER, dopamine reacts inappropriately. Dopamine is known for its effect in mood stabilization,[13] and when a D-MER mother's dopamine adjusts for prolactin, it does so either by falling too low, lowering too much, moving too fast or some other variance of the norm. Because dopamine stabilizes quite quickly after prolactin starts its climb,[14] the emotional reaction only lasts a couple of minutes. It also is felt emotionally before a mother physically feels her milk release because the neurotransmitters and hormones are moving faster than the milk does. By the time a mother is releasing milk, her dopamine has nearly finished its job and is normalizing again, as is the mother's mood.

This is the very basic guess about what is happening when a mother experiences D-MER. It is by no means certain, nor all inclusive. Other hormones or neurotransmitters may be at play. Also, what kind of inappropriate activity dopamine is taking is also not fully understood. Because supporting the

---

[13] Clin Neuropharmacol. 2005 Sep-Oct;28(5):228-37. Dopaminergic contribution to the regulation of emotional perception. Salgado-Pineda P1, Delaveau P, Blin O, Nieoullon A.

[14] A mathematical model of prolactin secretion: Effects of dopamine and thyrotropin-releasing hormone by Chontita Rattanakul and Yongwimon Lenbury

dopamine levels of a mother with D-MER seems to lessen her symptoms, it can be concluded that dopamine is the main culprit and that the levels are the "wrong kind of low". Neurotransmitters have the ability to act inappropriately in a variety of ways, which is why the guess of dopamine dropping too low, too quickly or too much in quantity of it is the best way to explain what is not known.

The Prevalence Of D-MER
There is often an assumption made that D-MER is rare among mothers, and this speculation may not be very beneficial to mothers with D-MER who often feel alone, isolated and like a "freak". Existing research and clinical experience has shown, repeatedly, that finding other mothers that have the same experience as she does reduces shame and isolation.[15] Isolating a mother further by classifying her experience as rare, is not likely to be helpful and it is far from certain or factual.

When considering the possible prevalence of D-MER, many things need to be kept in mind:
- How many mothers do not initiate breastfeeding (that may be predisposed to D-MER)
- How many mothers wean before their milk volume increases (when D-MER first starts to represent itself)
- How many mothers are predisposed to D-MER but wean for other breastfeeding struggles within the first couple of weeks (such as poor latching or breast infection)

---

[15] Shame and non-disclosure: a study of the emotional isolation of people referred for psychotherapy. by Macdonald and Morley

- How many mothers wean because they do not like the way they feel emotionally when breastfeeding and immediately wean (without ever knowing it was D-MER)
- How many mothers that do breastfeed with D-MER, and yet stay silent
- How many mothers are there that have come forward and made themselves known as mothers with D-MER.

Adding all those mothers together could show a very different picture of the prevalence of D-MER. Given the complexity of the phenomenon, the estimation of how common the experience of D-MER is, cannot even be guessed.

Predisposition To D-MER

It is not known why some mothers experience D-MER and others do not. It can be theorized that there could be some kind of breakdown in the way the neurotransmitters and hormones function for an undetermined reason. This could be concluded because there are mothers that may not have D-MER with their first, or first few babies, and then will have it with a future child. When this happens, it is almost a guarantee, it seems, that she will be affected by D-MER with any future breastfeeding experiences. There have been a variety of theories suggested, some of which remain viable explanations or starting points for future research. It does not seem evident that birth experience, birth medications or birth intervention affects D-MER. It does not seem that a history of mental health difficulties increases the risk of D-MER, nor does it seem to have a genetic component amongst family members. Medications or birth control do not seem to hold any influence. It does not seem to be apparent that HSP (highly sensitive people) are more susceptible to D-MER. It can affect mothers of any age group, westernized demographic or ethnicity. Whether a modern day diet, vitamin D deficiency or something else that goes against what is intended for a mother's body, anthropologically and biologically, is always a possibility. All the mothers that have been questioned about their D-MER are ones that are living a more westernized life. D-MER in third world cultures or indigenous communities has not been explored and remains unknown. If D-MER results from a breakdown of balance inside the body, modern and westernized health, lifestyle, genealogy, habits, diet and exposures could be something that comes into play with whatever may be causing a failure in the appropriate activity of dopamine in a mother with D-MER. It remains possible though, that D-MER is something that can happen, and has been happening, to some mothers across time. With the pattern of some mothers not having D-MER with first babies, but having it with all subsequent babies, this still alludes to some kind of eventual deterioration of the system. If not for reasons stemming from modern life, than perhaps simply for reasons of normal and natural biological wear and tear.

Commonalities Amongst Mothers With D-MER
Mothers on the support pages and forum for D-MER are hungry for explanations and correlations amongst them. Many women post informal surveys and inquiries about birth experiences, history of mental health problems, other family members that had D-MER, medications or birth control use, lifestyle, age, location, number of children, thyroid issues, medical history, general health status, history

of trauma or abuse, RH factor/blood type, certain personality types, prior diagnosis of personality and mood disorders, and more. In the initial informal surveying of D-MER mothers all these same inquiries were made. At this time, though, it is always possible to find another mother or a handful of mothers with similarities in any of these categories, there is no overwhelming pattern, marker or connection between the majority of mothers with D-MER.

Similar Phenomena

There have been some reports from people who are not lactating who resonate and relate to the way that D-MER is described and explained. It does seem that there are other instances of a very similar emotional experience that manifests in other situations.

There is a subset of women that relate an emotional experience, similar to how mothers explain their D-MER, when their nipples are stimulated, but outside of lactation. Where this has been casually discussed online it has been referenced as 'sad nipple syndrome'. These women talk about the sadness and hollow feeling in their stomach when their nipples are stimulated, most often during sexual activity. This dysphoric nipple stimulation does not appear to be a precursor to D-MER by any means, and women with D-MER are not prone to having dysphoric nipple stimulation experiences prior to lactation. These two experiences appear to operate independently of each other despite the similar feelings. The two have occurred in the same woman before, but this seems to be more coincidence than predisposition to dysphoric episodes.

Other women have come forward because, they too, resonated with how the feeling of dysphoria that is described within D-MER, but these were also not lactating women. They were menopausal women who became aware that they were about to have a hot flash, because they learned to recognize that right after a sudden and unexplained emotional drop of sadness and a hollow feeling in their stomach, they would then have a hot flash. This particular anomaly has not been casually or medically referenced by any name, but the occurrence of dysphoric hot flashes has been reported. None of these woman reported having D-MER during their lactations.

Other women have joined the conversation, because they too, though not lactating, recognized the way D-MER was described by its tell tale emotional signs. These women experienced an abrupt but brief feeling of similar D-MER like dysphoria in post coital and post orgasm occurrences. This condition is named post coital dysphoria and is currently being researched.[16] Some mothers with D-MER experience this, but like the dysphoric nipple stimulation, this seems to be a chance combination and not a connection.

There has been one case of a mother who had a late miscarriage, after 6 healthy live births and 6 normal lactations, who experienced D-MER symptoms for months after her dilation and curettage (D&C) and then, long after her milk supply dried up, she also experience the emotional

[16] Sex Med. 2015 Dec; 3(4): 235–243. Postcoital Dysphoria: Prevalence and Psychological Correlates Robert D Schweitzer, PhD,corresponding author 1 Jessica O'Brien, MA (Clin Psy.), 1 and Andrea Burri, PhD 2

phenomena post coital. In this case it points to being originally D-MER that then led or resulted in PCD.

There was a single report of a non-lactating woman with a seizure disorder who strongly identified with the description of D-MER as the kind of dysphoria she would feel prior to having a seizure.

It is likely that in all these instances that oxytocin, prolactin and dopamine are dancing their dysphoric dance. Why some experience it and not others is unknown. And these experiences are ones that do not go hand in hand, and do not indicate predisposition to one another. A mother may have D-MER, but not be troubled by nipple stimulation with she is not lactating. A woman may have dysphoric hot flashes, but she may have never had trouble breastfeeding. A woman may be prone to post coital dysphoria, but has never had an experience of dysphoric nipple stimulation. However, a few women report having more than one of these experiences. Why these experiences can operate independently as well as sometimes go hand in hand, is a matter for further investigation and research.

High Supply

A vast majority of mothers with D-MER reported having milk supplies that tend to be higher or oversupplies. Many of them have more forceful letdowns, more spontaneous letdowns, increased leaking and shorter feeding times. Milk supply volume is controlled by prolactin levels,[17] so it is very

---

[17] Blood and milk prolactin and the rate of milk synthesis in women Authors Cox DB, Owens RA, Hartmann PE

likely that there could be a correlation with mothers with D-MER being more susceptible to high milk supplies. Though these things are not interchangeable. There are many mothers that have high supplies and do not experience D-MER, and not all mothers who report having D-MER, feel that their milk supplies are high. There is a trend to high supply, but it is not consistent enough to draw many conclusions. Also, a mothers' interpretation of her own milk supply is subjective in itself. Many first time mothers with high supplies do not know anything differently. Moreover, a mother with a low supply may have one due to external factors such as a baby's insufficient milk removal or medications she is taking. But since the majority of mother's with D-MER report high supplies that border or cross the line of bothersome and hard to manage, it is noteworthy.

Thirst

Most mothers with D-MER report severe thirst when they experience the dysphoric episode. Medically speaking, extreme thirst is referred to as polydipsia and studies have shown that the dopaminergic neural systems do effect the intensity of polydipsia.[18] In the studies done thus far it is not conclusive of exactly how the neurotransmitters play a role in extreme thirst, but it has been shown that changes in thirst behavior may result from a change in the balance of activation of dopamine receptors. It is not uncommon for nursing mothers to experience some thirst when nursing, but D-MER mothers do most commonly report a strong and

---

[18] J Pharmacol Exp Ther. 1994 Nov;271(2):638-50. Polydipsia and dopamine: behavioral effects of dopamine D1 and D2 receptor agonists and antagonists. Mittleman G1, Rosner AL, Schaub CL.

overwhelming thirst. Though there is no conclusive evidence for how exactly this is being triggered by D-MER, it made be helpful for some mothers to know and understand that thirst is something that is increased when dopamine receptors are being negatively affected and the distribution and supply of dopamine is being blocked. In short, a mother with D-MER need not be confused by this experience and can recognize it as part of her D-MER, and keep water nearby when it is time to nurse.

Chapter Five
How D-MER Is Managed

D-MER does not have an evidence based treatment approach, as there has not been enough study and research done into the phenomenon. Based on anecdotal evidence, that low dopamine activity at time of the MER is the cause of D-MER, there have been some suggestions and ideas that may help ease D-MER. These come from medical professionals, as well as from experienced mothers with D-MER, and are generally safe for nursing mothers to try. Mothers with D-MER have also been able to recognize day to day tips and tricks to help them deal with their D-MER; noticing that aside from things can help to reduce the intensity of D-MER, there are also factors that can aggravate it.

What Can Make It Worse
Maternal self-reports suggest a number of issues that have been found to aggravate D-MER. While some of these are not always possible to avoid for the new mother, they can be

helpful to keep in mind for the mother and her support network.

Pumping

Whether directly nursing vs. pumping eases a mother's D-MER is a matter of personal position and preference, though it does seem common that D-MER is worse with pumping, especially when pumping two sides at once. As one mother accounted, *"I exclusively pumped with D-MER for the first 6 weeks due to baby's tongue tie. It's been snipped and now we're nursing, no pumping. I have not had those feelings at all while nursing."*

For mothers that find that their D-MER is worse when pumping, it is worth mentioning that the feel-good bonding hormone, oxytocin, is likely to be at higher levels when a mother is with her infant. This could help counteract, even if slightly, the intense dysphoria that a mother experiences with D-MER. One mother communicated, *"the pump was way worse for me. I was double pumping and I felt like I was drowning kittens. The worst kind of shame ever."* In cases where D-MER is worse when pumping, then pumping and stimulating both sides of the breasts is also likely to increase the intensity of the hormonal and neurotransmitter actions and cause dual pumping to be more emotionally intense. Another mother recounted, *"pumping is bad for me because I feel it isolates me more and my sadness intensifies."*

For mothers who find pumping easier than nursing, there are some speculations to possibly explain why this is. When a mother has her baby at the breast, milk is going to move more efficiently partly because a baby is more effective at the breast than a pump is. But in the case of pumping, the hormonal response to less effective stimulation may be lower, thus in theory less oxytocin and prolactin changes would occur in the body, perhaps also lessening the misaligned activity of dopamine in D-MER as well. Although this is purely theoretical, it is one possibility for the difference. Some other mothers have shared about how pumping was easier for them: *"Pumping was easier than nursing because I never had to manage a squirmy or fussy baby while trying to manage my own emotional state." "The desperation of the baby to latch and get milk makes me feel hurried and more stressed. Being able to take deep breaths and go slow with a pump is much better." "Pumping is easier than nursing because I connect these feelings of disgust and sadness to a machine rather than my baby." "I didn't have anxiety about pumping because even though the symptoms were worse, it was okay to loath the pump. When nursing my sweet babies, I had anxiety that I didn't feel happiness that other mothers felt when nursing."*

These two experiences (pumping being worse vs. nursing being worse) are at odds and the concrete reasoning is completely unknown, but the majority of mothers report at less emotional dysphoria when nursing their baby directly at the breast.

Nighttime
There are mothers that report that their D-MER is worse at night. One mother expressed, *"I've found at night that it changes, I'm wondering now whether it's because I tend to*

lay down to feed at night time with her because of reading about how some women have different experiences with different positions. At night I get suddenly fidgety and restless, I feel like my skin is crawling and like I need to just get away from it all." There may be a scientific basis for this. The circadian rhythm is partly influenced by the relationship of melatonin, norepinephrine and dopamine. "Results demonstrate a mechanism in which dopamine, normally increased at times of stimulation, can directly inhibit production and release of a molecule, melatonin, that induces drowsiness and prepares the body for sleep," explains Dr. McCormick. This means that in order for norepinephrine (which regulates the synthesis and release of melatonin) dopamine levels lower.[19] This may explain why D-MER mothers feel an increased dysphoric response to the MER at night. Like this mother said, *"I experience the sadness during the day, but it's not too horrible and I feel like I can deal. But nursing at night is becoming impossible. I don't enjoy it like I do in the morning and afternoon, and my milk doesn't let down, so it takes forever and I get no sleep."*

Sugar
Sugar is somewhat of a contradiction when it comes to dopamine and D-MER. Some mothers have reported that eating chocolate or carbohydrates can make a positive

---

[19] Sergio González, David Moreno-Delgado, Estefanía Moreno, Kamil Pérez-Capote, Rafael Franco, Josefa Mallol, Antoni Cortés, Vicent Casadó, Carme Lluís, Jordi Ortiz, Sergi Ferré, Enric Canela, Peter J. McCormick. Circadian-Related Heteromerization of Adrenergic and Dopamine D4 Receptors Modulates Melatonin Synthesis and Release in the Pineal Gland. PLoS Biology, 2012

difference with their D-MER. One mother wrote, *"eating carbs made D-MER less severe. I found this out when I tried to diet. I cut back on carbs and Gatorade and my episodes where horrific! They took my breath away and I couldn't move. As soon as I reintroduced Gatorade and ate more carbs the attacks weren't as debilitating."* This is understandable since sugars stimulate dopamine receptors in the brain.[20] But in order for sugar to sustain this, there needs to be a consistent source of it and sugar is burned through quickly, hence the term "sugar crash". One mother reported attempting to switch to a paleo diet (no sugars or grains), and stated her D-MER became much worse as a result. This would be because the body becomes dependent on the use of sugar to perpetuate dietary-induced dopamine dysfunction.[21] It would not be healthy to consider sugar, in the form of cane sugar or carbohydrates, as a sustainable treatment of D-MER. If sugar is looked at as a drug to the brain, as many experts do, it may be better for mothers to view sugar as something that can wreak havoc on the dopaminergic system. Though for a time D-MER may feel worse if sugars were cut out from a mother's diet, it may ultimately stabilize the natural levels of dopamine activity that a mother has, and help her assess her baseline of dysphoria more accurately.

---

[20] Neuroscience. 2005;134(3):737-44. Daily bingeing on sugar repeatedly releases dopamine in the accumbens shell. Rada P, Avena NM, Hoebel BG.

[21] Evidence for sugar addiction: Behavioral and neurochemical effects of intermittent, excessive sugar intake by Nicole M. Avena, Pedro Rada, and Bartley G. Hoebel

Caffeine

Caffeine is a similar quandary to sugar. Mothers report varying affects on their D-MER, some saying that it is worse and some saying that it is better. It could be similar to the issue of a sugar crash. Dopamine is stimulated in the brain by caffeine, by increasing dopamine signaling.[22] In theory this may ease a mothers experience of her dysphoria, but it could also make it feel worse as the caffeine wears off. By altering dopamine levels through various substances, that are short lived in the body, a mother will be more aware of the changes of intensity of her D-MER causing her to notice the worse MERs more readily. Some mothers share their experiences staying away from caffeine as follows:

"I notice that going off of coffee has eased up the intensity. When I have some caffeine it is way more noticeable." *"It's definitely worse for me if I have lots of caffeine, so I've been cutting back/weaning off caffeine."* *"I had more caffeine than usual yesterday and noticed D-MER was worse. I was a crazy person yesterday."* These experiences are very contradictory to these following testaments: *"I'm thinking back to pregnancy and the couple of weeks after my babies were born and I was having very little caffeine. Almost none. My D-MER was bad! Now, I'm having a lot of caffeine, more than I should be, and my D-MER is almost gone. I only experience D-MER during some letdowns and not all."* *" Caffeine helps decrease the severity of my symptoms."* *"Caffeine! Oh, my sweetest friend. Sometimes I feel like the only part of the day I feel totally normal is the*

---

[22] Caffeine increases striatal dopamine D2/D3 receptor availability in the human brain by N D Volkow,* G-J Wang, J Logan, D Alexoff, J S Fowler, P K Thanos, C Wong, V Casado, S Ferre, and D Tomasi

two hours right after drinking a cup of coffee while pumping. The constant dopamine dips are brutal, so the mini-lift I get from coffee is something I really look forward to." This last mother mentions the exact reason why caffeine could be of concern and ultimately less helpful, the dips as the caffeine leaves the system. A mother can weigh the options and decide what seems to be the best option for her in regards to caffeine.

Lack Of Self Care
There are three basic life influences that mothers frequently report making their D-MER worse. In the face of caring for a young baby, these can be hard to manage and prioritize but they are worth mentioning. Stress, dehydration and chronic fatigue are all thought to alter dopamine levels.[23] Not surprisingly, mothers with D-MER frequently report how much these things aggravate the intensity of their dysphoria.

Maternal accounts suggest that stress is a significant factor that plays a part in the aggravation of D-MER If a mother is already under duress when the MER is triggered, the

[23] Neuroreport. 2011 Jul 13; 22(10): 489–493. Sleep Deprivation Differentially Affects Dopamine Receptor Subtypes in Mouse Striatum. Miranda M. Lim,1 Jinbin Xu,2 David M. Holtzman,1 and Robert H. Mach2
Logo Neuroendocrinology. Changes in the Rate of Dopamine Synthesis in the Posterior Pituitary during Dehydration and Rehydration:Relationship to Plasma Sodium Concentrations. Alper R.H. Demarest K.T. · Moore K.E.

Differential Effect of Stress on In Vivo Dopamine Release in Striatum, Nucleus Accumbens, and Medial Frontal Cortex. Elizabeth D. Abercrombie, Kristen A. Keefe, Daniel S. DiFrischia, Michael J. Zigmond

dysphoria is going to bring her that much lower and make it feel much more intense than it would on a day when she feels less stress and pressure. A mother shared, *"I've been suffering from D-MER eleven months now, while nursing my twins. I have anxiety with each letdown. It is worse when I pump, and worse when I'm very tired or very stressed (which with twins, is a lot of the time)."*

Sleep is hard to come by with a new baby, and though chronic exhaustion and dopamine have a relationship, since sleep deprivation reduces dopamine D2/D3 receptor availability,[24] here too lies another basic emotional component; feelings are harder to manage, rationalize, accept and work through when one is especially tired. So for the sake of supporting dopamine levels as well as for better emotional coping, staying rested can help keep D-MER from feeling worse. One mother easily made this connection and stated, *"my capacity to deal with the strong emotions was just so much lower when I was exhausted (which was often). It made it really intense and harder to focus on getting past it."*

Aside from maintaining good hydration, some mothers find that drinking a cold glass of water during their first few letdowns of a feeding can help reduce some of the physical and emotional malaise of D-MER.

---

[24] Evidence That Sleep Deprivation Downregulates Dopamine D2R in Ventral Striatum in the Human Brain by Nora D. Volkow, Dardo Tomasi, Gene-Jack Wang, Frank Telang, Joanna S. Fowler, Jean Logan, Helene Benveniste, Ron Kim, Panayotis K. Thanos and Sergi Ferré Journal of Neuroscience

Medications

Some mothers have talked about how various hormonal birth controls and medications have affected their D-MER and either lessened it or worsened it. Reports about this are scarce and they vary in their content. Most breastfeeding mothers that talk about the mini-pill, which is an estrogen based birth control, state that it caused their D-MER to change slightly. Aside from birth control, any medications being used should be considered by a mother with D-MER and her healthcare provider, since the mechanism of D-MER is not fully understood and could be slightly affected in one way or another by a variety of medications/substances.

This can include galactagogues (herbs or medications that are used to increase milk supply), as many of these target the hormones of lactation. Domperidone is often prescribed to support a low milk supply. The drug itself is a dopamine antagonist.[25] This is how it can increase milk supply. Dopamine and prolactin (the hormone that makes milk) have an entangled relationship. Domperidone works by blocking the D2 receptor which allows for an increase in prolactin. This blocking of the D2 receptor could result in a further hormonal imbalance for a mother with D-MER that could potentially worsen or cause a dysphoric MER for some mothers. Any galactagogues could result in this for a mother that may have, or be at risk of, D-MER. This is because many of the drugs and herbs of this class effect and can alter the dopamine/prolactin balance of hormones inside of lactation. There is reference in a study published in Breastfeeding

[25] Domperidone, a new dopamine antagonist. M C Champion, M Hartnett, and M Yen

Medicine of a mother with D-MER that took the galactagogue Reglan (metoclopramide) to increase her supply, which in turn aggravated her D-MER.[26]

Invalidation And Isolation

Mothers who are not taken seriously by those around them report more severe D-MER and a harder struggle coping with it. Not only is the mother's knowledge about D-MER important to help her make sense of her experience, but the validation and recognition by her support people and care providers is just as crucial. Emotionally struggling in loneliness is a painful experience for any human, and mothers with D-MER have an especially unique challenge that puts them in need of connection, understanding, empathy and validation. Family, friends and partners can offer active listening and empathetic replies, they can make themselves present to help meet the mother's emotional and physical needs as well as giving her general recognition and validation of her experience.

D-MER And Other Emotional Challenges

If a mother has a history of mental health problems or a history of abuse she may struggle with D-MER more than other mothers. Indeed, people who have difficult emotional histories often tend to struggle with emotionally fraught situations, and in this way D-MER is no different. Because D-MER can be a vaguely familiar feeling that is so disturbing it becomes easy for mothers to wonder if it is because of

---

[26] Breastfeeding Medicine, Dysphoric Milk Ejection Reflex: A Case Series, Ureno, Tamara; Buchheit, Toni; Berry-Cabán, Cristóbal; Hopkinson, Susan

repressed memories or because of their particular emotional history. One mother voiced, *"I have randomly gotten D-MER like 'rushes' of terrible feelings for about 30-second intervals since I was maybe 6 years old. I thought it was some kind of repressed memory of sexual abuse, even though I have the most kind and loving family that would never, ever have done anything like that to me; finally, when I got the 'rushes' again while breastfeeding my first baby, I researched and found out about D-MER, and realized it really was not abuse, but an hormonal issue. I have had some degree of depression and anxiety most of my life as well, so the symptoms all seemed to fit. It helped the awful D-MER feelings immensely to know that it was chemicals, rather than repressed memory or something I was doing to myself to cause it. Now, I'm just hoping I do not get it, or can at least manage it better, when my next baby is born."* Other mothers who are aware of their difficult pasts and need to navigate D-MER through breastfeeding after sexual abuse. Penny Simkin, author of 'When Survivors Give Birth', writes, *"for many survivors, some of the greatest challenges in the postpartum period occur with breastfeeding."* D-MER is going to increase this challenge two-fold. Though mothers do not get D-MER because they were sexually abused or because of a traumatic birthing experience, a mother may feel a reminiscence of an earlier time in her life during her D-MER. Though this is not indicative of a psychological response to breastfeeding.[27] When a mother experiences D-MER, the emotions she feels may cause her to remember those upsetting times in her life, but the experiences themselves are not triggering the dysphoria in her MER. The emotions she experiences with D-MER may mimick how she felt during those times, and trigger old memories, emotions and sensations. The MER itself creates the dopamine drop in a mother's body. With a dysphoric MER it is going to make a mother feel negatively regardless of her past life experiences, but since D-MER causes a very distinct bad feeling, it may be what seems like a familiar bad feeling for a mother.

What Can Help With Correction Of D-MER: For Mothers

Many mothers with mild or moderate D-MER find that they do not feel compelled to find medicinal correction for their D-MER with medication or herbs. This is especially true when mothers feel stable in mood otherwise. Most often having their D-MER validated, recognized and understood is enough to give mothers enough peace of mind that they can continue nursing without risk of premature weaning. For those who do not feel the need for medical intervention, there are simple practices that most mothers with D-MER tend to implement to help ease the discomfort that they do feel throughout their nursing sessions (see figure 18).

---

[27] Maternal experiences of embodied emotional sensations during breast feeding: An Interpretative Phenomenological Analysis: Marcelina Watkinson, DClinPsy (Dr), Craig Murray, PhD, DHealthPsy (Dr), Jane Simpson, PhD, DClinPsy (Dr) Division of Health Research, Furness College, Lancaster University, Lancaster LA1 4YG, United Kingdom

Self Care

Prioritizing self-care with a new baby can be almost a laughable idea. Lack of sleep, no time to shower and meals eaten standing up are common and expected for new mothers. Prioritizing rest, staying well hydrated, maintaining low stress levels, getting exercise and consuming a healthy diet are hard even without a new baby. These basics of self-care, however, are especially invaluable to a mother with D-MER. If a mother has the support system that allows her to prioritize herself in these ways, she will find her D-MER to be much more manageable. Many mothers express that D-MER is much worse when sleep deprived, under undo stress, and dehydrated. Simply enough, this is not surprising. Any negative emotional experience that we encounter on a day to day basis is ultimately much harder to manage when we are not feeling resilient. One mother admitted, *"If I am already having a hard day it feels like D-MER is hitting me when I'm "already down" so to speak."* It seems that these self-care staples are either that much more helpful (if taken care of) or harmful (if neglected) to a mother with D-MER. Aside from the healthy balance that good self care brings, dopamine levels can be affected with added stress and poor sleep.

Drinking Ice Water

A large number of mothers report that actively drinking a glass of ice water during their dysphoria makes it more manageable. The reason for this can only be guessed at. Cold water showers are often cited for having positive effects on dopamine,[28] though reference or research into drinking cold water are not found. Regardless of the lack of evidence based information, there is plenty of anecdotal reports of the positive benefits of drinking ice water to ease D-MER, and it is by far the most often suggested tip on D-MER boards for mother to mother support: *"Drinking ice cold water seems to help me through it. Maybe it's a distraction but it works."* *"When I'm sitting I try to have water or any drink with me and drink during the attack."* *"Drinking ice water while it happens seems to help me some."* *"I feel my D-MER is worse when I forget my water bottle."*

Distraction

Mothers tend to lean in one direction or another when getting through an episode of dysphoria, using either mindfulness or distraction. The more popular choice between the two though, is distraction. A mother wrote, *"distraction helped; white-knuckle clutching my phone and scrolling through Facebook or anything."* This can be an excellent tool, and many mothers find great relief in being able to ignore their emotional disruption. This is initially counter intuitive. When having a negative emotional reaction, it is generally known that getting curious about our feelings often results in a better understanding of ourselves, and therefore also increases the ability to meet our own needs. Many mothers initially do this before they understand that D-MER does not demand any self examination. With D-MER, the emotional reaction is not because of the phone call

---

[28] Eur J Appl Physiol. 2000 Mar;81(5):436-42. Human physiological responses to immersion into water of different temperatures. Srámek P1, Simecková M, Janský L, Savlíková J, Vybíral S.

she just had with her mother-in-law, it is not because she is worried about her third graders performance in math and it is not because she feels guilty that the house is a disaster and she is ordering pizza for dinner, again. It is an emotional reaction that has nothing to do with her or her life. Therefore, the permission to disconnect from herself can be a gift. Using a smart phone, the internet, Facebook, any social media, Netflix, a phone call, texting, TV, a video game, reading or listening to an audio book can be great tools. Some mothers, especially with severe D-MER, find that it is best to stay away from distraction techniques that are more social or relationship oriented. This is because in very sensitive cases of emotional tides, a mother may coincidentally experience dysphoria right after she hits "post" or "send", only to find herself unnecessarily overthinking her interaction. If this is the case, sticking to Candy Crush and binge watching Orange is the New Black may be a safer form of distraction.

Mindfulness

A less common choice, but one that can work very well for some mothers, is engaging in mindfulness. To be clear, this is different from dissecting one's feelings and emotions in order to control them, rationalize them or understand them. At its core, mindfulness is about acceptance and awareness. The skill of sitting with uncomfortable feelings is an approach that is often used in meditation. Here it is emphasized that the act of letting thoughts and feelings come, exist and then move on can be a therapeutic way of accepting the impermanence of emotions. It can be a good skill for life in general and even more helpful with D-MER. Just like distraction, it gives a mother the room to not try to understand, make sense of or fix her feelings. It allows her to just feel the wave of emotion without labeling, judgment or thought; and then move on. A mother recounted, *"finding out what it was, how it worked and that I was not the only one with it helped enormously. I found 'growling' to myself through the letdown to get me through to the other side helped, then using cognitive behavioral therapy techniques immediately following to remind myself that the negative feelings were not real, were only temporary and were chemically induced helped me get back on an even keel."* While D-MER does not have anything to do with a mother or her life, the feelings may offer a window to exploring those aspects that it triggers. For some mothers with D-MER, it triggers the areas where there was already a vulnerability. So in that sense D-MER does link to her and her beliefs about herself. Mindfulness may help her understand why D-MER feels connected to those real life experiences.

Counseling

Though D-MER is physiological, it is very emotionally upsetting and mothers can feel very distraught and isolated in their circumstance. Some mothers find comfort and validation in being able to talk about their experience with an understanding and educated therapist. This would be someone who could help a mother understand that the feelings of D-MER are not manifesting due to issues to fix, pick apart or heal from. Coping skills of awareness and mindfulness can be shared and learned in this kind of environment, alongside gaining a broader vocabulary, awareness and intelligence around her emotional experience. A mother can use such opportunities to talk about other areas of her life that are affected by D-MER, her

94

disappointment with not having the expected breastfeeding experience or to learn how to better control her responses to the emotional episodes, even though she cannot control the emotional reaction itself. A mother who feels that, she is left with unsettling emotional concerns and issues even after D-MER has corrected, may benefit from counseling. Mothers who are nursing with D-MER, combined with a mood disorder or difficult life circumstances would benefit from considering mental health support as well.

Self Education

There are two helpful ways in which a mother with D-MER can educate herself to handle her experience of D-MER more easily. The first is for her to learn what there is to be learned about D-MER and to stay connected to information, stories and updates about D-MER itself. Educating herself about the phenomenon may increase her confidence when making sense of and sharing her experience with those around her. Education supports a mother to have a stronger feeling of empowerment and a sense of peace about what she is going through. Education about D-MER has the power to ease a mother's discomfort and to make D-MER slightly more tolerable. The second way a mother can self educate is by expanding her emotional vocabulary and by learning about various cognitive functions and distortions. Many mothers have a hard time separating themselves from the dysphoria and find that cognitive dissonance and cognitive distortion can take place as a tool for the mind, as it tries to avoid uncomfortable emotions. If a mother educates herself about these psychological processes/defenses (there are as many as 50 cognitive distortions) she may be able to find a better understanding of herself and her experience.

Connection And Sharing

Mothers with D-MER find that sharing, talking, story-telling and connecting with others to be invaluable in seeing her through her journey. Whether is it having a reliable outlet for expressing her feelings and sharing her struggles with someone who helps her feel heard and seen, journaling in a private journal, sharing on online message boards or talking to other mothers with D-MER on support group pages; all these things help a mother feel stronger in dealing with her D-MER.

Self Correction

Waiting for D-MER to self-correct is something that all mothers that struggle with D-MER do. Wondering if and when it may correct, and if she can make it that long, is much of a mother's thoughts. It can be helpful to a mother to think of her D-MER journey in 3 month blocks. Often mothers with mild D-MER find self correction by 3 months, if not, then by 6. Mothers with moderate D-MER often find relief between the 6 and 9 month mark. Being able to take breastfeeding in these more manageable 3 month goals can be helpful. A mother can ask herself if she can make it three months. If the answer is yes, than she can set aside further reevaluation until she has made it that far. Instead of wondering each day if she can make it and whether and if D-MER will correct soon, she can evaluate and examine these questions once every three months. Alternatively, some mothers may take better comfort and find more control in a simple day to day approach, asking herself if she feels if she can make it through today. Though this seems to be a stark contrast to the 3-month evaluation mindset, it serves the same purpose of shrinking down the overwhelming big picture of 1-3 plus years of breastfeeding with D-MER.

Ways To Support Dopamine Levels

There are a variety of naturally occurring things that help support dopamine levels that could be safely tried by a mother with D-MER. This section comes with a big disclaimer around health because so much of the content below is speculative and inferred from other known information. The speculative and anecdotal solutions are being included because it is how future research can emerge, but it comes with a bit of a warning. These suggestions are generic in nature, and may or may not be targeting D-MER's root cause.

- Vitamin D plays a role in releasing neurotransmitters. Vitamin D3, particularly, is associated with an increase in dopamine levels. Furthermore, vitamin D deficiency is known to decrease the availability of a dopamine gene that is responsible to the development of dopaminergic neurons.[29] This is being studied more in relationship to Parkinson's Disease (PD), which is a disease characterized by the loss of dopaminergic neurons, and in a case report it

---

[29] eNeuro. 2016 May-Jun; 3(3): ENEURO.0122-15.2016. Published 2016 May 19. Vitamin D3: A Role in Dopamine Circuit Regulation, Diet-Induced Obesity, and Drug Consumption1,2,3 Joseph R. Trinko, Benjamin B. Land,Wojciech B. Solecki, Robert J. Wickham, Luis A. Tellez, Jaime Maldonado-Aviles, Ivan E. de Araujo, A. Addy, and Ralph J. DiLeone

was shown that an increase of vitamin D lessened symptoms of PD.[30]

• Similarly, sunlight provides a role in healthy dopamine levels. There is research that connects sunlight exposure to the number of dopamine receptors.[31] It is known that sunlight can affect serotonin levels, but the amount of light exposure may also influence dopamine.[32] It is thought that that it takes at least 30-60 minutes per day to get a dopamine increase from sunlight.[33] Biologically we are designed to be outside a good amount of time, being exposed to the sun on a daily basis. So it would make sense that a minimal amount of sun exposure may cause a variety of neurotransmitter and vitamin deficiencies.

• Vitamin B6 (pyridoxine) is essential for normal brain development and function, participating in the process of

[30] Role of Vitamin D in Parkinson's Disease by Khanh Lương * and Lan Nguyễn

[31] Prog Neuropsychopharmacol Biol Psychiatry. 2011 Jan 15;35(1):107-10. Sunshine-exposure variation of human striatal dopamine D(2)/D(3) receptor availability in healthy volunteers. Tsai HY1, Chen KC, Yang YK, Chen PS, Yeh TL, Chiu NT, Lee IH.

[32] J Psychiatry Neurosci. 2013 Nov; 38(6): 388–397. Dopamine and light: dissecting effects on mood and motivational states in women with subsyndromal seasonal affective disorder. Elizabeth I. Cawley, MSc, Sarah Park, MSc, Marije aan het Rot, PhD, Kimberley Sancton, BSc, Chawki Benkelfat, MD, DERBH, Simon N. Young, PhD, Diane B. Boivin, MD, PhD, and Marco Leyton, PhD

[33] Top 16 Proven Health Benefits of Sun by Josh Finlay

making dopamine.[34] B-vitamin complex is a treatment that makes some sense with regards to why D-MER has become a more prevalent problem, as nutrition deficiency in our culture is a very common issue and vitamin B is an important one for neurological health. Taking a full B-complex supplement while breastfeeding is safe and this supplement can be found in the vitamin section of the grocery store.

- Magnesium has the possibility of having a positive impact on dopamine and mood stabilization. There is some speculation that the rise of depression rates is due to magnesium deficiencies.[35] With the theory that D-MER is possibly due to a biological breakdown, vitamin and nutrient deficiency is certainly an area to consider. Studies suggest that magnesium has a positive effect on the dopaminergic systems of the brain.[36] Magnesium supplements are available over the counter, and magnesium levels can be tested by a health care professional.

---

[34] Nutrients. 2016 Feb; 8(2): 68. Published online 2016 Jan 28. doi: 10.3390/nu8020068. B Vitamins and the Brain: Mechanisms, Dose and Efficacy—A Review. David O. Kennedy

[35] Psychology Today, Emily Deans M.D., Evolutionary Psychiatry, Magnesium and the Brain: The Original Chill Pill, Posted Jun 12, 2011

[36] Prog Neuropsychopharmacol Biol Psychiatry. 2009 Mar 17;33(2):235-42. Evidence for the involvement of the monoaminergic system in the antidepressant-like effect of magnesium. Cardoso CC1, Lobato KR, Binfaré RW, Ferreira PK, Rosa AO, Santos AR, Rodrigues AL.

- There is a body of evidence that points to a connection between gut health and brain health. Gut health refers to the balance of good and bad bacteria in the gastrointestinal track. Antibiotics can have a damaging effect and probiotics can restore balance. Research is indicating that gut bacteria can influence anxiety and depression.[37] Additionally, gut microbes have the ability to produce hormones and neurotransmitters.[38] Improving gut health is a very simple solution for a mother with D-MER to try. Mothers can work with a health care provider that is knowledgeable in this area to investigate the nutritional options for improving gut microbes therapeutically. These can include changes in diet, probiotics, and prebiotics.

- Dopamine is made up of the the amino acids tyrosine and phenylalanine.[39] Foods that increase these amino acids are eggs, turkey, chicken, cottage cheese, pork, whole milk, plain yogurt, granola, oats, wheat germ, dark chocolate, soy products, fish, peanuts, almonds, avocados, bananas, cheese, lima beans, pumpkin seeds, and sesame seeds. A mother with D-MER could include more of these in her

---

[37] When Gut Bacteria Change Brain Function; Some researchers believe that the microbiome may play a role in regulating how people think and feel. By David Kohn

[38] J Med Food. 2014 Dec 1; 17(12): 1261–1272. doi: 10.1089/jmf.2014.7000 The Gut Microbiome and the Brain by Leo Galland

[39] J Nutr. 2007 Jun;137(6 Suppl 1):1539S-1547S; discussion 1548S. Tyrosine, phenylalanine, and catecholamine synthesis and function in the brain. Fernstrom JD1, Fernstrom MH.

diet in order to support the production of dopamine in her body.

- Fava beans, also known as broad bean, faba bean, horse bean, field bean or tic bean, contain levodopa. Though recent studies show that the consumption of fava beans is not effective for severe dopamine related condition such as Parkinson's, fava beans do result in higher plasma levels of dopamine[40] and it could help support dopamine levels enough to improve D-MER. The young fave bean pod and the immature (green) beans inside the pod contain the greatest amount of levodopa, and the mature, or dried bean, the least. Three ounces (about 84 grams or ½ cup) of fresh green fava beans, or three ounces of canned green fava beans, drained, may contain about 50-100 mg of levodopa.[41] So because of the lower levels of levodopa in mature beans, the beans would need to be young green fava bean, not matured beans. If a mother is taking any other supplements or medications she should consult a qualified botanical prescriber before using fava beans, and she should make sure all prescribing doctors know about adding them to her diet and research the option carefully first. Because of the potency of fava beans they should not be used in conjunction with taking a prescription for D-

---

[40] Am J Clin Nutr. 2013 May; 97(5): 1144–1150. Published online 2013 Apr 3. An increase in renal dopamine does not stimulate natriuresis after fava bean ingestion1,2,3 Emily M Garland, Tericka S Cesar, Suzanna Lonce, Marcus C Ferguson, and David Robertson

[41] Scientific Society of Vegetarian Nutrition. Fava Beans, Levodopa, and Parkinson's Disease by Kathrynne Holden, MS, RD

MER. There is not much known about this option and consulting with a nutritionist would be advised. Like some of the other speculated nutritional options for D-MER, it is possible that fava beans could be an effective and safe solution for a mother with D-MER.

- DHA is the omega 3 that has the most positive effect on dopamine, and it may increase endogenous dopamine levels.[42] DHA can be found in fish oil supplements, fish, some omega 3 supplemented foods, as well as in breast milk. Something to consider, if a mother is comfortable with it and has an excess of milk, is to go ahead and receive the extra DHA by drinking her own milk. Otherwise, buying quality DHA supplements to take may help ease a mother's D-MER.

- Exercise regulates and increases dopamine in the brain.[43] Studies imply that it requires regular exercise and that it is most likely more than 30 minutes of aerobic exercise at a time is needed to achieve the benefits. In the busy life of taking care of a baby, it is understandable that making time for this commitment would be challenging. Nonetheless, it bears mentioning as a possible way to ease the severity of D-MER.

---

[42] Biomol Ther (Seoul). 2012 Mar; 20(2): 152–157. Effects of Docosahexaenoic Acid on Neurotransmission
Kazuhiro Tanaka, Akhlaq A. Farooqui, Nikhat J. Siddiqi, Abdullah S. Alhomida,and Wei-Yi Ong

[43] Neurobiol Dis. 2003 Jun;13(1):1-14. Regulation of brain function by exercise. Sutoo D, Akiyama K.

- There is increasing evidence suggesting that meditation can support healthy levels of dopamine.[44] If a mother commits to learning how to meditate, and she is able to make it a daily practice, it would be possible to improve the presence of neurotransmitters, including dopamine. "There is evidence in particular that mindfulness meditation is capable of increasing signaling in areas of the brain involved in emotional regulation and control of attention. It is the increased activity in these regions that has been found to increase the release of dopamine."[45] With the demands of motherhood, meditation may not be a plausible commitment for some mothers as, to achieve the dopaminergic benefit, the practice of meditation needs consistency and time. But their may be mothers who have a history of meditation practice that can be reestablished, or the interest and ability in establishing a new one.

- Massage therapy results in a significant increase of dopamine.[46] Though it is not possible to lay down on a massage table before every feed, it is possible that regular treatments could ease a mother's D-MER for a short time. Perhaps mothers could also have a partner or support person offer soothing massages on a regular and frequent

[44] J Psychiatry Neurosci. 2011 Mar; 36(2): 75–77. Biologic effects of mindfulness meditation: growing insights into neurobiologic aspects of the prevention of depression. Simon N. Young, PhD

[45] http://mentalhealthdaily.com/2015/04/17/how-to-increase-dopamine-levels/

[46] Int J Neurosci. 2005 Oct;115(10):1397-413. Cortisol decreases and serotonin and dopamine increase following massage therapy. Field T, Hernandez-Reif M, Diego M, Schanberg S, Kuhn C.

basis.

- Tyrosine and phenylalanine are the amino acids that dopamine is made of and,[47] in addition to occurring naturally in some foods, are available as a dietary supplement. When a consulting nutritionist was approached about this treatment, it was said, *"while adequate precursor levels of tyrosine and phenylalanine are necessary for dopamine production, more building blocks will not necessarily result in more dopamine unless protein deficiency was a contributing factor to the dopamine deficiency."* It is possible that a protein deficiency could be an aggravating cause of D-MER but it is unknown what D-MER's triggering factor is, so these supplements may not help. If a mother is interested in pursuing this avenue than it is desired that she does so under the advice of a nutritionist that she proceeds with caution since, with all protein supplements, a mother will want to be careful to watch the dose.

- Cytidine diphosphocholine or CDP-choline is a supplement that is made to mimic another substance that is made in the body that, from studies done for Parkington's Disease, appears to increase dopamine

---

[47] J Nutr. 2007 Jun;137(6 Suppl 1):1539S-1547S; discussion 1548S. Tyrosine, phenylalanine, and catecholamine synthesis and function in the brain. Fernstrom JD1, Fernstrom MH.

levels.[48] There is no readily available information on this supplement, so a mother would need to further investigate it with a health care professional and talk to a care provider about its use.

- Some mothers report that they have had good success with acupuncture. A mother would want to request from the acupuncturist a treatment that would regulate dopamine (preferably in the nucleus accumbens part of the brain.) There have been some studies done on this kind of acupuncture and an educated acupuncturist should be able to reference them in order to know the specific acupuncture points.[49]

- Out of the suggestions above, the ones reported by mothers that seem to have made the largest positive impact on D-MER are vitamin B complex, magnesium and vitamin D.

Talking To Medical Professionals

Talking to medical professionals about D-MER can be intimidating for mothers at first. Not only is it important

---

[48] Neuropharmacology. 1984 Dec;23(12A):1403-6.
Cytidine(5')diphosphocholine enhances the ability of haloperidol to increase dopamine metabolites in the striatum of the rat and to diminish stereotyped behavior induced by apomorphine. Agut J, Coviella IL, Wurtman RJ.

[49] PLoS One. 2011;6(11):e27566. doi: 10.1371/journal.pone. 0027566. Epub 2011 Nov 22.
Acupuncture enhances the synaptic dopamine availability to improve motor function in a mouse model of Parkinson's disease. Kim SN1, Doo AR, Park JY, Bae H, Chae Y, Shim I, Lee H, Moon W, Lee H, Park HJ.

and helpful for a mother to get the support and validation that she needs, but it is also a rare opportunity to help educate those in the medical profession about D-MER.

Many mothers with D-MER have had poor experiences talking with care providers about D-MER, a mother reported, *"after reading about D-MER my symptoms were cut in half. But after sharing about my feelings with the lactation consultant at the hospital, she told me I "must be an aggressive mother". I felt like crap. So, I thought I was just crazy. Listening to others talk about it and knowing I'm not alone has been the biggest help!"* Another mother mentioned, *"D-MER kind of spread to my whole day because in those few seconds I thought about real worries that I had, so then it was hard to step out of that dark zone, and now I think I'm a bit depressed. I'm sure that D-MER can lead to depression, mostly if you do not have any medical support, like in my case. The doctors and psychologist did not even know what it was so they thought it was part of postpartum depression, depression, anxiety, and so on. That convince me even more that I cannot breastfeed for a long period, because I will not get medical help and I feel like it is inhuman being forced to deal with this alone; it's too strong. And they insist like I am crazy but that I must breastfeed, using all kind of guilt trips, and using my child to make me feel bad. That's dangerous because I know that you can even feel rejection towards your child due to all the pressure doctors and midwives put on breastfeeding, they just think I'm a crappy mother and do not care about my struggles. I guess the main point with D-MER is that you end up feeling like a bad mother, and feeling guilty, depressed, etc. Then, instead of getting help from medical professionals, you just receive accusations, criticism and pressure."* Experiences and fears such as these can be intimidating to a mother who wants to reach out for support and help.

A mother will benefit from keeping in mind that she is likely to know more about what she is experiencing than her healthcare provider. Being able to speak from a place of knowledge and confidence will aid her. As a patient it is easy to feel intimidated in the face of a care provider; especially as a new mother who may already feel out of her element. While many medical professionals pride themselves in having a broad and research informed knowledge base, there are still significant knowledge gaps in the research and clinical fields. This also holds true for research and clinical activity in lactation. If a mother can speak with patience as well as self-assurance it may help her to not feel invalidated or bullied when working with a health care professional that may lean to the more skeptical or dismissive side of things.

Bringing along information about D-MER will help both the mother and provider as they talk about D-MER. This can be in the form of the handouts that are available about D-MER, as well as reference information from Google Books and Google Scholar. These resources are all listed on the resource section of this book. There are many lactation texts that recognize D-MER, as well as a handful of case studies and academic research. This is the kind of information that helps medical professionals be more understanding and receptive of the emotional experience that a mother with D-MER is attempting to communicate. It can also help to have an International Board Certified Lactation Consultant (IBCLC) as an advocate if needed. An IBCLC will be more likely to be familiar with D-MER, and if not, is also more likely to become more curious than dismissive about what a mother is communicating to her. Once a mother feels supported by her LC, if she then finds herself dealing with a resistant/hesitant doctor, she can request the doctor contacts her LC so that she can have a care giving team that is on the same page. Alternatively, a mother's LC can contact and work with the mother's doctor in order to better support the mother from a united and understanding place.

If a mother is intimidated by an uncertain or hesitant medical caregiver, it may be helpful to keep in mind that medical professionals often welcome continued education, and this can be an opportunity to help provide that. If a mother feels unable to articulate or make herself understood to her care provider, it is possible that bringing along an advocate, such as a partner, parent or friend, to support the conversation may reduce some of those concerns.

It's heartrending to hear about mothers who are easily disregarded by health care providers who do not take the time to listen to mothers about their feelings and experiences. This is especially evident when a mother approaches the health care provider as a self educated woman who has new and insightful information to offer. It is still far too frequent for women to be dismissed for their emotional experiences, to not be taken seriously and to be invalidated by those in the health care community. A mother voiced, *"I mentioned D-MER to my doctor today. He basically scoffed at me and said "I have been working with breastfeeding women for 45 years and there is never* *anything new with breastfeeding just different interpretations of it".* Then he suggested I switch to bottles and said that nothing else can be done. I was a bit astounded by his ignorance and unwillingness to listen."* Women and their emotions have a long history in medicine as being a troublesome nuisance and have been labeled and maltreated for decades of medicine. It will only be through determination and volume that this trend turns towards the desire to hear and understand women and their emotional make-up and struggles. Breastfeeding mothers speaking up about D-MER is an integral part of helping make that change.

Ultimately, if a mother finds that anyone in her healthcare team is more damaging and neglectful to her D-MER situation, it would be wise for the mother to search out a different care provider that can offer her the kind of support she needs.

What Can Help With Correction Of D-MER: For Medical Professionals

D-MER is not a "diagnosable condition" at the time of writing this book. It is not found in diagnostic referencing, it does not have a diagnostic code and it does not have a standard course of treatment for medical caregivers to reference. This makes it hard for mothers and medical professionals to know how to best help or alleviate D-MER. There are some suggestions that have helped some mothers, and these are made based on the preliminary conclusions about the mechanism of D-MER. From the suggestions that follow, the mothers that have tried medication have had the most success with bupropion and those that have tried a herbal remedy, the most success has been found by using Rhodiola.

Medication

This section has been co-written with Diane Wiessinger, MS, IBCLC

If there is concern from a care provider regarding the use of these drugs in a breastfeeding mother it is suggested that <u>Dr. Thomas Hale's book, "Medications and Mothers' Milk"</u> be consulted.

Bupropion, the active ingredient in Wellbutrin, is the most likely solution for D-MER at this point as it seems that anything that supports or increases dopamine is likely to improve D-MER. There are a few other medications that increase dopamine but they are not sustainable for use all day every day. Since some mother's D-MER is so severe that she does not feel like she can continue without a sustainable option of relief, it is good to be able to offer something that may help and is sustainable for everyday use.

To offer a brief understanding of how bupropion works; hormones are chemicals that are released by cells into the bloodstream, stimulating or blocking activity in other cells. Neurotransmitters are chemicals that are released by nerve cells (neurons), stimulating or blocking activity in other neurons. A signal travels electrically within the neuron, out to its very tip, releasing a neurotransmitter that now has to cross only the tiniest of gaps in order to stimulate the neighboring neuron. The neurotransmitter quickly fastens itself to receiving points, called receptors, on this neighboring neuron. Any "leftover" neurotransmitter is taken up again by the transmitting neuron. A drug that keeps a transmitting cell from taking back its released neurotransmitter is called a "reuptake inhibitor".

Neurotransmitters work faster than hormones, just as electricity travels faster than a river. That's probably why D-MER mothers feel the dysphoria before their milk starts to flow. The milk release reflex is triggered within their brains by neurotransmitters that have already done their job by the time their hormonal partners have reached the breast to release milk there.

The brain is fairly well protected from blood contaminants by the "blood-brain barrier". That means that raising the blood's level of a chemical does not necessarily raise the brain's level, so we sometimes have to be sneaky when the neurotransmitters we want to affect are inside the brain itself.

Dopamine is both a hormone and a neurotransmitter. It is probably its role as neurotransmitter within the brain that matters in D-MER. This is where the tricky part comes in. Since no one can squirt extra dopamine into the bloodstream and have it cross the blood-brain barrier to reach the brain, if an increase in brain dopamine levels is desired then these are 4 ways to achieve that: 1) make the brain increase its own output of dopamine, or 2) make the brain release a chemical that the receptors will accept as if it were dopamine, or 3) keep the transmitting cells from taking back left-over dopamine, so that there will be more available for the receptors to keep accepting, or 4) increase the number of receptors.

Bupropion (Wellbutrin) is a "dopamine reuptake inhibitor," which means it allows an individual's own dopamine to be used more completely, essentially increasing their dopamine levels. There are other dopamine reuptake inhibitors, and there are "dopamine agonists," which fool the receptors into behaving as if they've been given dopamine. However, at this point bupropion has the best track record as a medication for breastfeeding mothers. It's also familiar to physicians, who have probably prescribed to breastfeeding women before, so it is often viewed as a safe option to try.

A mother with D-MER does not need a high dose. A typical dose for depression is 150mg to 300mg per day, often given in a once a day extended release pill. A 300mg per day dose is sometimes used to help quit smoking. We suspect that these levels are unnecessarily high for many D-MER mothers.

A mother may consider starting with 100mg time release pills, and beginning with one pill per day. If that seems inadequate, she can work her way up slowly, always working with the advice and supervision of her doctor about how and when to increase or decrease the dose. Extended release pills must not be broken to change dosage.

A side caution to consider is that any drug that raises dopamine levels will lower prolactin levels, so dopamine reuptake inhibitors and dopamine agonists are not generally advised for breastfeeding mothers. This is because they could lower her milk supply. However, based on very limited observations it is possible that D-MER mothers may be resistant to the drop in supply that other mothers might experience. If D-MER mothers are starting with slightly less dopamine (and thus slightly more prolactin) than usual, a small increase in dopamine should simply "level" them, the way thyroid medication just brings a mother's thyroid hormones back into her normal range. Nonetheless, it needs to be recognized that bupropion is off label use for D-MER, and it would be important to watch for a decrease in supply if bupropion is used.

With regards to the safety of this drug in a mother's milk, the amount of bupropion that the baby gets is no more than 2 percent of the mother's dose.[50] If the baby has started solids, the amount of drug he gets will be even lower. Blood levels of bupropion were undetectable in the babies' blood when 10 mothers took 150mg per day for 2 days and then 300mg for another 5 days. There were no side effects noted. There is single report of seizures in a 6-month-old whose mother had taken 150mg per day for 4 days. She discontinued the drug and continued breastfeeding with no further effects. It is unknown if the single incidence was connected to the drug certainly, or not. But low transference of the drug is what studies have shown.

Many breastfeeding mothers have taken bupropion at the usual antidepressant dose of 300mg, and a dose for D-MER is only one third that high to start with, but it is still a prescription drug. Discuss its appropriateness for the mother with the doctor and pharmacist.

---

[50] Thomas Hale. Medications and Mothers' Milk. 14th edition

It is important to note why other antidepressants will not help with D-MER. Most of the antidepressants typically prescribed to breastfeeding mothers are SSRIs. Serotonin does not seem to be the neurotransmitter that needs targeting with D-MER. The SSRIs may help any generalized or postpartum depression that a mother may have in addition to D-MER, but mothers report that they have not helped with D-MER.

Some mothers may not be advised to use bupropion. If a baby is very young or D-MER symptoms are mild, a mother might want to wait before seeking a prescription. However, if she is thinking of weaning, or has an older baby (a mother and doctor can define for themselves what "older" means in each case), a low-dose prescription may be a possible option. It's very early in the game for specific recommendations so talking with a pharmacist and doctor about it, and taking into account the age of the baby and severity of symptoms is paramount. Remember that a very low dose is probably all that is needed. Also advised is that a mother looks over the suggestions for natural treatments and lifestyle changes for further help before considering a prescription.

Herbs

For all herbs it is recommend that a mother works with an herbalist about safety and dosage. Also, referring to the book The Nursing Mother's Herbal by Sheila Humphrey is advised. Lastly, as with all herbs, it is important that they be attained from a reputable source.

- Rhodiola, also known as roseroot or golden root, is a herb that helps rebuild dopamine in the brain stem, rhodiola compounds stimulate the release dopamine.[51] This has been experimented as treatment for D-MER on a small scale with good results, and is the most likely natural remedy to have a lasting impact on D-MER. Because of its strength and because it acts as a MOAI (monoamine oxidase inhibitor) it should not be used in conjunction with a prescription for D-MER. Though this is the most widely used herb to treat D-MER, there have been no official studies done or published on its effectiveness to treat D-MER. It has been studied, however, to treat anxiety and depression.[52]

- Chasteberry (also called vitex berry) is an herb that, at high doses, can truly affect the dopamine system in the brain.[53] It inhibits prolactin secretion and increases dopamine activity with regular use at high doses. Because of its strength is should not be used in conjunction with taking a prescription for D-MER. This also means at a high dose it is an antigalactagogue and a dopaminergic so the milk supply needs to be considered with this herb. Chasteberry takes one month or more to reach its maximum effectiveness. This is an herb that is harder to

---

[51] Nordic Journal of Psychiatry. Volume 61, 2007 - Issue 5. Clinical trial of Rhodiola rosea L. extract SHR-5 in the treatment of mild to moderate depression

[52] The Journal of Alternative and Complementary Medicine. A Pilot Study of Rhodiola rosea (Rhodax®) for Generalized Anxiety Disorder (GAD). Alexander Bystritsky, Lauren Kerwin, and Jamie D. Feusner. The Journal of Alternative and Complementary Medicine. March 2008, 14(2): 175-180

[53] Botanical, chemical, genetic, and pharmacological studies of Vitex agnus-castus L. 2011 by Donna E. Webster

find and is not available at most health food stores.

- Ginkgo is an antioxidant that can increased dopaminergic transmission.[54] It has been shown to increase blood flow to the brain and supports many cognitive functions. Like many things that increase dopamine, Ginkgo can also lower prolactin levels, so milk volume should be evaluated and monitored. It is advised to start at a lower dose of 120 milligrams, but doses as high as 600 milligrams can be taken.[55]

- Cowhage, also known as Mucuna Pruriens, is a possible natural solution. Mucuna Pruriens seeds are a natural source of Levodopa. Levodopa is a dopamine precursor. Cowhage has been used to treat Parkinson's symptoms as many as 4500 years ago by Indian physicians practicing traditional medicine. The benefit of cowhage seeds is due to the fact that these seeds contain 3-4% levodopa.[56] According to WebMD, "the appropriate dose of cowhage depends on several factors such as the user's age, health, and several other conditions. At this time there is not enough scientific information to determine an appropriate range of doses for cowhage. Keep in mind that natural products are not always necessarily safe and dosages can

[54] Br J Pharmacol. 2010 Feb; 159(3): 659–668. The Ginkgo biloba extract EGb 761® and its main constituent flavonoids and ginkgolides increase extracellular dopamine levels in the rat prefrontal cortex. T Yoshitake,1 S Yoshitake,1 and J Kehr

[55] Ginkgo Biloba WebMD

[56] Northwest Parkinson's Foundation. Is natural dopamine better than Sinemet? By Monique L. Giroux, MD

be important. Be sure to follow relevant directions on product labels and consult your pharmacist or physician or other healthcare professional before using." Though supplements can be found in multiple places online, mothers are advised to consult a nutritionist for dosing instructions.

- Though no studies have been done, Evening Primrose Oil (EPO) is thought to increase the availability of levodopa in the body. Levodopa is converted to dopamine in the brain. In the online health communities EPO is recommended to alleviate Parkinson's symptoms. EPO is a common and low-risk supplement that a mother could try without much concern.

Validation And Education

The biggest gift, help and support that a health care professional can give a mother with D-MER is help, support and acknowledgment. Mothers with D-MER are often uncertain and doubtful of their own experience and truly want it to be recognized and affirmed by a medical professional. Mothers who are courageous enough to share their experience with a care provider and meet with resistance and skepticism find themselves even more emotionally vulnerable than before. For a mother who does not need, or is not interested, in medication or herbal correction, recognition is significant source of treatment for her affliction. For a care provider that is hesitant to prescribe or treat a mother with D-MER in a medical sense, starting with recognizing the mother and the mothers situation may remedy a mothers severity to a significant degree. One mother eagerly posted, *"I have insurance that covers lactation support and we have a perinatal unit with lactation consultants. I recently reached out to one regarding D-MER to see if she had any suggestions and to my amazement she did! I kept a log for 3-4 days of when I felt it, time of day, which side, what I was doing/feeling. She reviewed my data and suggested a few natural things: B complex, increased DHA (at least 250mg- my vitamin only has 200 mg per tablet), increase water, and Ginko Biloba. We are going to check in after a few weeks, but I am noticing a small difference in that I do not feel the absolute low. I feel the sad/hollow feeling but it's not this gut wrenching going-to-cry feeling. So if you have access to someone like this, try it out!"* This mother used some natural remedies, but mostly found a high amount of encouragement and rejuvenation just by working with a supportive healthcare provider.

Chapter Six
How Support People And Professionals Can Help

Lactation and lactation support is about relationships; between mother and baby, between mother and support people, between mother, baby and support people. A meeting with a healthcare provider who is educated about D-MER, can offer a truly valuable gift of validation and relief to a mother having such experiences.

Being Able To Recognize A Mother With D-MER

Most mothers start to notice D-MER between 5-7 days postpartum. Many do not connect it to letdown until 2-4 weeks postpartum. If a health care provider is going to ask a breastfeeding mother questions about D-MER, it is best to time it right. It will help to wait until things are well established and a mother has actually had a chance to notice anything that may not feel right. The ideal time is 10-14 days postpartum, unless it is suspected the mother is at risk of weaning sooner, possibly due to D- MER. The language a mother uses is noteworthy. The way a mother describes her D-MER experience helps aid in its recognition. Mothers with D-MER often use very similar language and words. Very rarely will there be only a simple utterance of "I do not like breastfeeding". In fact many mothers with D-MER like breastfeeding aside from their moments of dysphoria. When a mother begins to open up about the negative feelings she is having at the time of milk release, her description is likely to involve a number of the following words and phrases:

- hollow
- intense
- feels like
- seconds
- stomach
- rush
- overwhelming
- minutes
- fade away
- feelings
- before letdown
- loss of appetite
- wave

- sudden
- pit in stomach
- negative
- gut-wrenching
- throat tightening
- visceral

These are the most frequently reoccurring words when mothers talk about their D-MER (see figure 15).

Questions To Ask To Help Mother's To Share About Possible D-MER

(See figure 20)
- How is breastfeeding going?
- How is it different then how you expected it to be?
- Do you get those stereotypical "warm fuzzies" when you nurse? Not all women do.
- How have you been feeling?
- Any hints of anything that looks like the baby blues or PPD?
- Do you like nursing?
- How does breastfeeding make you feel?
- Do you ever sit down to nurse and suddenly realize how tired you are and how much work all this is?
- Does it ever surprise you how emotional becoming a new mother can make you?
- Have you ever stopped to notice how you feel right before and during letdown? Some moms experience such different things!
- Have you ever heard of dysphoric milk ejection reflex?

If A Mother Has D-MER

There is an easy acronym to remember when working to support a mother with D-MER which is called VASE (see figure 16).

- Validation: Validate a mother's feelings and struggles as significant
- Acknowledgement: Acknowledge that D-MER is physiological
- Support: Support her in her situation and decisions
- Education: Encourage the mother in education and finding support for D-MER

A number of mothers with D-MER initially think that they are crazy. This is a recurrent word that mothers use when they first find out about D-MER. Mothers exclaiming, *"I am so glad to have this information, I thought I was crazy"*, is a frequent post on the D-MER.org support page. This is why validation is the first step in supporting a mother with D-MER. Letting a mother tell her story and share her feelings; while empathizing with her struggles goes a long way in helping her feel less shameful and make better sense of her experiences. It is extremely powerful for a mother to hear from a professional that her situation has a physiological basis that is out of her control and is not her fault. Affirming her that she did not do anything to cause her D-MER and clarifying that it is a biological anomaly reduces distress and frees up her resources to make sense of her experiences. From there a mother may begin to talk about how she feels and make a truly informed decision about handling her D-MER. Supporting a mother in this processing is paramount. She may seesaw back and forth between weaning, toughing it out, and considering some kind of treatment. Approaching her with curiosity during this stage, listening for cues for what seems to be most important to her and encouraging her in following her gut all contribute to the mother's own formulation of the issue and offers a direction for her own solution to emerge over time. A mother does not need to make any decisions right away, and simply letting her have some time with the new knowledge of D-MER can bring her further peace and understanding. This is where encouraging a mother for further self education about D-MER and pointing her to sources of support and connection comes in. Many mothers find solace in the knowledge of D-MER and the company of other mothers that are also going through it. Most importantly, a health care provider who simply knows of D-MER and can affirm a mother in her situation can go further than anything else.

Questions To Ask If D-MER Is Suspect
Below is a list of questions that a clinician can ask a mother who may be experiencing D-MER. Accompanied with them is a rough outline of what a mother may answer and how indicative of D-MER it may or may not be.

Can you explain what kind of feelings you experience?
A mother will usually focus on two things, her emotional reaction (using words that are synonymous to either sadness, anxiety or agitation) and also the visceral sensations that she has in her stomach. Though a mother may think (or explain) this as a physical discomfort, such as nausea, usually either on her own (or with guidance) a mother with D-MER will be able to express that it is some kind of emotional churning and discomfort that happens in her stomach.

How long do the bad feelings last?
Generally a mother is going to state that the feelings last for a few moments or minutes. She may say that they come in waves throughout the feeding. Very rarely will a mother say that the feelings last throughout the whole feeding and if that is the case, it is possible that something else is going on. In cases where mothers have severe D-MER and a supply of milk that produces many MERs close together, it is possible that she may not feel a break in her D-MER experience until the letdowns slowdown or space more widely.

When do you notice the negative emotions?
If a mother has connected her feelings to milk release, then she may state that she feels them right before milk release. If, however, the mother is unaware of when her milk letdowns occur because she does not feel physical signs, she may find the feelings to be random or sporadic throughout her day or only when nursing. A LC can show the mother how her baby's sucking pattern changes with a letdown, and the mother can watch to see if her feelings manifest 30-90 seconds before the baby's sucking pattern alters for the greater flow of milk.

How do you feel during the rest of the day?
Unless a mother also has PPD, then she should report that she feels fairly normal and stable except for during a D-MER episode. Even mothers with PPD can recognize that, though they feel depressed and low most of the time, that D-MER is much different and causes them to suddenly crash and feel worse, returning to their "normal" level of depression after the D-MER is over.

When did the feelings first start?
Mothers with D-MER first notice their feelings within the
first month of lactation. If the emotions started later than
that it would be good to inquire about new medications, a
change in nursing patterns, major life stressors, a change in
habits such as caffeine or nicotine or other inquiries that
could have changed to alter the mother's normal dopamine
activity. If the unrest with nursing started after 9-12 months
of age, then exploring the possibility of nursing aversion
would be an appropriate step to take.

*Do you have these feelings with just nursing or with
spontaneous letdowns and pumping?*
Most mothers with D-MER will experience D-MER with all
three; especially those with severe D-MER. There are
mothers, however, that may experience it just with pumping,
or just with nursing, or not at all with spontaneous letdowns.
The answer to this question is most indicative and helpful
when a mother does have D-MER with all three kinds of
letdowns.

Do you feel anything in your stomach when it happens?
The word nausea when used with D-MER is not quite
accurate and can result in mothers who just experience the
physical complaint of nausea with letdown to call it D-MER.
Mothers with D-MER may use the word nausea as to
simplify her experience and for lack of a better word. As a
care provider it is important to tease out the actual
experience of discomfort that the mother has in her body.
Often mothers will talk about a sense of unease in their

stomach and it is helpful to avoid the word nausea since the two letdown phenomena are so frequently confused.

Do you have any other feelings (physical or emotional) other than the feeling in your stomach when it happens?
A mother with D-MER really only uses language that would describe an emotional experience; similar to someone talking about how they felt after an upsetting event. For instance: if someone was to recall an aggressive verbal confrontation thrust upon them, it may be explained that they felt shaky and sweaty, their heart rate increased and their heart thudded in their chest; but this would be described as happening because they felt fearful, shameful and exposed. Likewise, a mother will focus on her emotional feelings with D-MER, and perhaps explain some further physical sensations that came from those. But D-MER does not have distinct physical markers in its manifestation.

Worries About The Effect Of D-MER On The Baby
A mother may worry that her preoccupation of her feelings is not good for the baby. She may feel like it is getting in the way of bonding. Indeed, on some level, it is true that D-MER may interfere with the mother staying more present through a feeding experience. However, many breastfeeding mothers are distracted and multitasking while breastfeeding, and most mothers do not get locked in with her baby during every feed, soaking up every oxytocin induced attachment experience. All mothers talk to other family members, use their phones, computers or TVs, make lists, plan dinner, and do other various tasks while breastfeeding. Anthropologically a breastfeeding mother would not be able to spare the time of sitting still and resting with her baby during every feeding,

so it is quite normal for a mother to be otherwise distracted while feeding her baby. The mother with D-MER is not denying her baby in any way by being less than present with nursing. Additionally, mothers who are aware of their absence due to D-MER may sometimes overcompensate for their lack of presence during breastfeeding in other aspects of caring for their baby. There are many other opportunities during the day for a mother to adore, stroke, talk to and coo at her infant, when she is not experiencing D-MER. Reminding a mother of this can be helpful.

Some mothers may worry that the baby is picking up on the mother's feelings, and sensing her discomfort and mood change. This can concern the mother that there is a transference of anxiety or distress to the infant. Though there is a concern about poor attachment being formed between mother and child if the mother has PPD,[57] this is due to the fact that the mother's continual low mood and struggles with depression can negatively affect her availability to care, nurture and bond with the baby. Mothers with D-MER have no problem offering their child comfort, attentiveness and care though, as her low mood is not a problem outside of her short D-MER episodes. A recent study has found a correlation between chronic stress in the

---

[57] Paediatr Child Health. 2004 Oct; 9(8): 584–586. Depression in pregnant women and mothers: How children are affected

home and childhood development,[58] but again, D-MER is quite different than a chronically stressful home environment. A mother concerned about her infant absorbing the mother's own emotions would be concerned about the baby's level of empathy, since "feeling another's feelings" is about one's ability to empathize. It has been shown that as early as 10 months of age, an infant can show a sympathetic response, but only to visual cues[59], not to innate empathetic instinct. This kind of transference would take a level of emotional awareness and intelligence. Research tells us that the empathic response and ability to hold another person's mind in mind, is one that develops over time, peaking in mid-life.[60] A mother who is concerned about her baby reacting to her emotional distress can work on her own emotional regulation as well as her ability to pick her emotional responses, even though the emotional reactions cannot be controlled. A mother can feel internally anxious without disruption of those around her with anxious or erratic behavior; it is the responses she chooses that are more likely to upset those around her, and this could include her baby.

---

[58] GENOMICS. Epigenetic Vestiges of Early Developmental Adversity: Childhood Stress Exposure and DNA Methylation in Adolescence. Marilyn J. Essex, W. Thomas Boyce, Clyde Hertzman, Lucia L. Lam, Jeffrey M. Armstrong, Sarah M. A. Neumann, Michael S. Kobor

[59] Psychology Today. Christopher Bergland. Empathy Appears in Infancy but Varies by Age and Gender

[60] Psychology Today. Christopher Bergland. Empathy Appears in Infancy but Varies by Age and Gender

Mothers with D-MER have also showed a higher concern about the stress hormone, cortisol, being in her breast milk in higher levels because of D-MER. The concern that mothers are expressing is the fear that, chemically, the feelings of D-MER could have a possible negative effect on her baby. There is research on the cortisol levels in breastmilk and that the presence of them do influence a baby's growth and behavior.[61] But the research is not indicating that this is a bad thing. Biologically the triad of mother, baby and milk are acting in the way it was designed, and science is not jumping to conclusions about the presence of cortisol in milk, either. One journalist wrote about the study, *"Increasingly, studies are showing that a mother's milk, in one way or another, helps to shape her child's behavior and temperament, and may deliver useful information about the environment she's growing up in. Perhaps my milk was sending my daughter a message: Here's what you need to know about the world. Act accordingly."*[62]

Lastly, there is breastfeeding folklore and an old myth about how negative or strong emotional feelings can make the milk turn sour,[63] and though this is not a common obstacle to

---

[61] Hormones in Mother's Milk Influence Baby's Behavior by Katie Hinde, Department of Human Evolutionary Biology, Harvard University

[62] When Stress Comes with Your Mother's Milk; Stress hormones in breast milk may help prepare us for a turbulent world. By Jena Pincott

[63] The Folklore of Breastfeeding by Marie Walters. Saddleback College

encounter as a lactation consultant in educated communities, it is one that can be encountered still among minorities and lower income mothers. This false folklore is worth keeping in mind when working with mothers with D-MER. A statement about how a mother's emotional state does not affect the quality of her milk could be helpful for some mothers to hear.

Concerns About Premature Weaning

Mothers with D-MER may have initial breastfeeding goals that may seem overwhelming or unreachable once they are in the midst of struggling with D-MER. A mother explained, *"it is just discouraging to keep breastfeeding when these feelings happen at every feeding. I look forward to weaning my son so I can enjoy life again!"* Mothers can hit various weaning thresholds that may cause them to wean earlier than they initially had hoped to (see figure 17). The experience of D-MER can be a slippery slope from discouragement to giving up, triggered as simply as a mother not liking the way she feels when breastfeeding. In the beginning this can be a confusing time for a mother who has yet to understand what is happening to her. It then becomes easy for a mother to begin projecting her feelings onto herself; beginning to believe something is wrong with her, that she is doing something wrong, or that she is the only one that feels this way. Since D-MER can often manifest with feelings of shame, these thoughts or beliefs only feed her self-doubt further. When breastfeeding is generally painted as such a pleasant and bonding experience and because it is natural, it is often mistaken for something that does not involve challenges and a learning process. Thus if a mother has never heard of anything like what she is experiencing, she is likely to begin feeling isolated and alone. Feeling lonely is never a healthy atmosphere for someone who is struggling and in need of support and understanding. If a mother is generally proactive, educated and has access to resources like the internet, then it is likely that she will go in search of answers at this time. Thankfully for that small subset of women, there are answers readily available and can alter a very hard situation into something more manageable through peer support. But many mothers do not have such an advantage. Often, if a mother is brave enough to speak about her concerns to another (like a friend, sister, or partner) who may have never experienced or heard of D-MER, she may not find the validation that she was hoping for. If she speaks to a health care provider, it is very likely that it may be a medical professional who has not been educated about D-MER yet, and their responses can be experienced as dismissive by the mother. Not uncommonly, misguided care providers have misdiagnosed D-MER as PPD and consequently prescribed medications for a condition that the mothers don't have. Over time a mother may feel increasingly alone and misunderstood, making her less resilient to cope with the emotional surges. Her self directed emotions can then feel oppressive and problematic, ultimately spilling over into other parts of her life. At any point one or many of these things could be enough to tip a mother over her own weaning threshold and cause her to give up much sooner than she intended or wanted to. A mother reported, *"I stopped after 6 months because I could not deal with D-MER anymore. I have two older children and had started to experience panic attacks. It was still a difficult decision to make, but I went completely back to normal a week after stopping. I have no regrets."* It is undeniable that mothers and babies are switching to formula sooner than desired because of D-MER, and that this is putting babies under unnecessary health risks. For this reason education, support and management of D-MER is necessary.

How To Advise A Mother With D-MER
Mothers with D-MER think and talk about weaning much more frequently than other breastfeeding mothers. Most breastfeeding mothers consider weaning during certain and specific times. These times often occur: 1. in the beginning of their journey 2. during the times of initial struggles 3. when their baby is older and they are thinking about going back to work 4. the end of the first year 5. with a nearly self weaning toddler. But mothers with D-MER may ruminate and think about if and when to wean throughout their whole breastfeeding duration. As a lactation support person, this can be hard territory to navigate. For some mothers with D-MER, it is such an invasive experience that it is seriously discoloring not only their breastfeeding experience but can seep into other parts of her life. It can bring up uncomfortable memories that are associated with some of the feelings of D-MER, it could cause her to project her emotions onto those around her, it may make her feel like she is not bonding with her baby, it could keep her in a place of continually questioning herself and in extreme cases it may cause her troubling thoughts of self harm or suicidal ideation. Every woman is going to have her own threshold of how much of this she is able to handle and where her limit is. It is important to encourage her to keep breastfeeding if that is what she wants, but it is also important to give her validation and support if she chooses to wean. As a counselor

or consultant this is an important time to utilize counseling skills and techniques.

Finding out what a mother's initial breastfeeding goals were, before D-MER, is the best starting place. It is also good to evaluate how much the knowledge and education of D-MER helped ease her experience. Those with severe D-MER do not find as much relief in that as mothers with mild D-MER do. Helping a mother explore various coping strategies and investigate any medical or herbal remedies can also be of support. Questions that guide her to the future may give her hope, by inquiring as to whether she feels like she can make it to the next 3 month marker. It is impossible for a care provider to know the depth of the mother's experience or struggle. Offering platitudes and trite sympathy can seem disconnecting and unsupportive to a mother. Empathy, genuine support and validation with plenty of room given for the mother to make her own choices will help empower her in a way that is more likely to extend her breastfeeding duration.

The Sensitive Issue Of Weaning

For the majority of mothers with D-MER it is a situation that does not require weaning. Every mother would benefit from being in an empowered position to choose what feeding method is right for her and her family, and there are many challenges and situations that cause mothers to choose to forgo breastfeeding. But D-MER is manifesting in mothers who have already established breastfeeding with the intent of breastfeeding their babies. For a mother to wean despite this choice, because of D-MER, is highly unfortunate, yet, some mothers with D-MER are choosing to wean or shorten the duration of breastfeeding. One concern about D-MER is the negative connotation it holds towards breastfeeding in a society where breastfeeding has been painted as a beautiful and pristine gold standard. In the developed world, breastfeeding rates had been steadily declining since the early 1920's and, after hitting a low of 22% in 1972, have climbed back up.[64] As of 2016 initiation rates in the US were at 81%.[65] Formula companies were held somewhat responsible for the low rates of breastfeeding in the 1980's before the WHO code changed the regulations that limited the access that formula companies had to marketing to mothers. This does not change the fact that formula companies still are able to target mother's vulnerabilities, marketing towards mothers who have babies with sensitive stomachs or difficult sleeping patterns that could be "fixed" by the newest kind of formula. The concern of formula companies using D-MER as a marketing tool to mothers is a valid fear among breastfeeding proponents. This is one reason why there is careful language around whether or not weaning is a viable solution for a mother with D-MER.

There are still many issues in the world of formula vs. breastfeeding; the most current one being mothers' guilt for not choosing "the best". As advocates for breastfeeding have been working to increase the rates of lactation for the health of mother and child, it is true that some methods chosen

---

[64] The American Society for Nutritional Sciences. The Resurgence of Breastfeeding at the End of the Second Millennium. Anne L. Wright and Richard J. Schanler

[65] 2016 Breastfeeding Report Card, CDC.

have had less than desirable effects and increased mothers' guilt is among them.

There is also an increase in the understanding that breastfeeding is the norm and therefore formula is the experiment. In this case the language such as, "breastfeeding reduces the occurrence of childhood diabetes"[66] is less true than the statement of "formula increases the risk of childhood diabetes". In this way, the "breast is best" campaign has over idealized what is, in fact, just normal. Breast is normal. In this context, the "benefits" of breastfeeding are in fact simply human norms and the use of formula is showing that those health norms are compromised.

With emotions running high, increasing concerns about the long term safety of formula, mom-guilt on the rise, the separation of formula feeding moms against breastfeeding moms; the issue of weaning can be a sensitive subject. One mother reported, *"I had moderate to severe D-MER with my last child, and I am glad this information exists online. However, I have one serious criticism of how most of the information is presented: I do not think it is helpful or appropriate to insinuate that the appropriate course of action is always to continue to breastfeed. Stating that formula feeding is supposedly "more risky" than all other treatment options (including taking a prescription) is very one-sided and, at best, does not reflect the full extent of the*

---

[66] Exclusive breastfeeding to reduce the risk of childhood overweight and obesity. Biological, behavioural and contextual rationale. WHO technical staff

scientific debate on the effects of breastfeeding vs. formula feeding in the developed world. In any case, without wanting to get into a discussion of breastfeeding, it is clear that weaning your child is a 100% effective way to end D-MER with no risk to the mother (and, as many researchers would argue, no discernible risk to the baby as long as there is access to formula and safe water). Of course, every effort should be made to develop and research treatment options for D-MER that are compatible with breastfeeding, as many mothers want to breastfeed very much. No woman should have to stop breastfeeding before she is ready. However, this is a very personal decision that depends on how a woman feels about breastfeeding, how severely she is affected by her D-MER, and how she feels about other options available to her (personally, I would definitely wean before taking a drug for a condition that can easily be resolved by weaning). No one but the individual mother can weigh these factors and decide which steps are appropriate for her. I would respect the information about D-MER a lot more if it were able to present all possible treatment options, including weaning, in a neutral way and trust women to make the right decision for themselves. Weaning is simply one option among several for women who suffer from D-MER."

The best way to handle it may be to say that while D-MER is not an excuse to wean, it is sometimes a valid reason to wean, just like any unresolved breastfeeding challenge can be. Lactation support people's main goal is to meet the mother where she is and to support her goals and ultimately her choices. Lactation consultants cannot ethically consider weaning a "treatment" for any breastfeeding problem, including D-MER. It is however, a result that can sometimes arise from any breastfeeding problem. In this way, some mothers themselves may choose weaning as a solution to D-MER and a lactation care provider can help her through her transition and the difficult feelings surrounding her decision. But a lactation consultant will first pursue the goal of a happy and healthy breastfeeding dyad if the mother wants the help, and in the field of lactation where the risks of formula are just as studied and understood as the risks of medication or herbal solutions; continued lactation will be supported and encouraged whenever possible. As lactation consultants continue to do their job in this way, it is also the job of the mother to know herself, her baby and the needs of both. Societal pressures about parenting decisions have a large impact on a mother's instinct, and in turn, the choices she makes. A mother who decides to wean because of any breastfeeding problem has the right to her choice as much as a mother who decides to continue to breastfeed despite breastfeeding difficulties.

Chapter Seven
Building Awareness

Until D-MER is something that is better researched and understood, there are limited options of how women can continue to find the support, answers, validation and help that they need. However, the one thing that everyone can do is raise awareness. With the internet often at our finger tips, with mothering communities and with the access to obstetricians, lactation care givers, pediatricians and nurses available to new mothers, there are many options for sharing information and educating others. It can take courage to do so. With so many that are unfamiliar with D-MER, it can be easy to be met with skepticism or resistance to new information. This is particularly true in the medical community, where many medical professionals are under pressure, from themselves as well as the wider public, to know everything there is to know.

Why Is D-MER So Unrecognized

D-MER is "new", or is it? After being first named in 2007, D-MER has been openly talked and recognized since at least 2010. Women have, of course, experienced it and struggled with it since before then, though for how long, it is not currently known. It is not known whether there is something in the modern day lifestyle or exposure that is causing a hormonal breakdown or if this phenomenon has been experienced by mothers throughout many generations. Lactation, as a science, is new itself and it has a complicated history.[67] Animal milk has been used as a breastmilk substitute as early as 2000 BC and clay feeding vessels for babies date back to the same time. By the time of the industrial revolution, when technology allowed for easier food preservation, many women were working outside of the home and science began to try to duplicate breastmilk. Breastfeeding rates significantly declined at this time. It was not until the 1970's, when Le Leche League sought to renormalize breastfeeding, and until the 1980's when

---

[67] J Perinat Educ. 2009 Spring; 18(2): 32–39. A History of Infant Feeding. Emily E Stevens, RN, FNP, WHNP, PhD, Thelma E Patrick, RN, PhD, and Rita Pickler, RN, PNP, PhD

formula marketing became ethically challenged, that breastfeeding rates slowly started rising. During this major loss of normal infant feeding practices, much of the innate breastfeeding knowledge that women had collected themselves over the centuries, was lost as well. When women were helping women, before there were doctors, lactation consultants, breastfeeding self-help books and lactation texts, the knowledge of breastfeeding was shared orally through generations and within communities. The struggles and complications of breastfeeding were understood and addressed within the knowledge these women held from collective years of supporting themselves and one another through the feeding of their infants. It is utterly possible that the knowledge of "bad feelings when breastfeeding" was something known and understood by women; women who were not writing lactation texts or publishing case studies. Another major consideration to make about why D-MER has not been openly discussed sooner, is the stigma around emotional problems. For example, even though the first documentation of emotional disturbances after childbirth can be traced back to 700 BC, it was not until the 1980's that postpartum depression was added to the Diagnostic and Statistical Manual of Mental Disorders (DSM).[68] This stigma around emotional difficulties emerged when information about D-MER was first being presented to the community of lactating mothers. Women were expressing that they were indeed scared to talk about their feelings with letdown. Once they felt safe and supported they admitted that they had not been talking about it or telling anyone; they had been keeping it a secret. For a time D-MER was referred to as

---

[68] A History of Postpartum Depression by Katherine Abalos

"breastfeeding's best kept secret", for this very reason. The secrecy around the experience, often resulted in maternal feelings of shame and when women feel ashamed, they often see silence as their only choice. Without the mothers talking about it, the care providers could not recognize it; and thus, it remained a hidden experience. It took time for emotional wellness and mental health to hold less stigma in society, as well as the first 100 or so courageous mothers to come forward, for D-MER to be recognized and hold any weight in the medical community. In the field of lactation there are dozens of brilliant professionals working to bring new information to the field, helping with issues such as low milk supply, infant bonding, mammalian response, abnormal breast anatomy, hormonal imbalances, breastfeeding with illness, the effect of medications and more. These people are not just working to do basic problem solving for mothers, but are working to bring evidenced based information to the study of human lactation. This is exactly what the slow work and understanding of D-MER is about; the process of bringing new information into the light for further research and understanding. This being said, the validity of D-MER is still questioned among many health care providers who may hold a conservative standpoint with regards to advances and new discoveries in research and clinical practice.

Sharing The Story

Mothers have a commonality after birth, and that is the desire to share their story. The telling of their narrative is a passage into motherhood as well as being an aid on the processing of the experience. It is very common for a new mother to share her story and have the women around her share theirs in kind, no matter how many years have since passed. This exchange and active participation in connecting over experiences is not only a valuable tool for mothers with D-MER in their own journey, acceptance and validation of their struggles, but can also be vital to spreading the information about the phenomenon. A mother with D-MER will benefit from working to free herself from any shame or embarrassment about her experience with D-MER. This can be hard when so few are familiar with it, just as it used to feel much more shameful for a mother to admit to or talk about her PPD. But mothers with D-MER are pioneers for shining light on the issue of D-MER and have an opportunity to use their voice to ease the journey of those who come after them.

Elevator Speech

It can help to speak on the subject of D-MER from a place of confidence, with nearly an air of assumption that one's audience is aware of the experience. If and when it becomes apparent that the listener is unfamiliar with D-MER, it can be of benefit to the speaker to have an "elevator speech" prepared about what D-MER is. An elevator speech is a clear, brief message about a particular topic and enables the communication about what D-MER is, how it affects a mother and what possible mechanisms are responsible for it. Elevator speeches are typically about 30 seconds, the time it takes people to ride from the top to the bottom of a building in an elevator. An example of an elevator speech about D-MER would be:

"D-MER is the acronym for dysphoric milk ejection reflex, which is a condition that can affect some lactating women that causes the mother to have a sudden and intense negative emotional reaction when her milk lets down. It happens with every milk release and it is thought to be caused by inappropriate dopamine activity when a mother's prolactin levels start to rise. It is still not very well understood, and more research is needed, but it can be very upsetting and disruptive to a breastfeeding mother, especially since she has a stable mood and feels normal except when experiencing the roller coaster of sudden emotional drops so often."

A video of a D-MER elevator speech on YouTube can also be found. Using this method for either a brief mention of D-MER or to open the door to further explanation or a deeper sharing of one's story can be a great tool when talking to those around a mother, in her family, circle of friends or in mother's groups.

The Internet
Blogging is a great tool for mothers to share their story, not only for its therapeutic value, but also for raising awareness. Even if someone does not have their own personal blog, guest writers are often welcome on already established blogs. Taking the time to write out one's own story and then exploring platforms where sharing it would be possible, can be an effective tool in spreading awareness.

Message boards are usual sources for finding other mothers who may be sitting in silence with their concerns about their feelings during breastfeeding. So many mothers are afraid to speak and admit how they feel. Thus, first sharing freely about one's own struggle with D-MER can help other mothers to find the help, information and support that they need. D-MER would not be as recognized as it is today if it had not been for a single post on a breastfeeding message board that helped finally bring silent mothers together.

Topic submissions or article submissions to online magazines are often sought after and a mother with D-MER may find that if she writes up her unique and particular experience with D-MER, there may be some online sources that would be interested in posting it. There are several articles about D-MER on online magazines out there, but each one offers a different perspective and individualistic outlook on the phenomenon and how it can affect a mother and her family. A mother does not have to be a writer herself for this avenue either, as many online magazine authors are frequently on the prowl for new interesting content.

The Media

Seeking out main media sources is often as easy as petitioning news or human interest resources online. Many news and human interest programs have websites that offer online forms for submitting suggestions for future coverage. This is a tool mothers can use to petition more major media outlets. Local or national news stations and reputable talk shows may be interested in the newness and uniqueness of D-MER if enough mothers come forward offering the resources and opportunity for their coverage.

The Medical Community

Educating medical professionals, aside from one's own individual one, is a distinct opportunity. Almost all doctor's offices, care facilities, hospitals, mothers' programs and the like, have training days and in-service days that are used for continuing education as much as they are used for interoffice updated policy trainings. If a mother can pair up with a member of staff, then the two may have an opportunity to give a short presentation about D-MER to the entire caregiving staff to share the information and to help educate about D-MER.

Further Case Studies

If a D-MER mother is working closely with a medical professional that is interested in publishing opportunities, a case study is the simplest and most straightforward route to do so. Nurse practitioners, obstetricians, lactation consultants and others may respond favorably to a mothers offer to be the subject of a case study. If a mother's care provider expresses explicit interest in a mother with D-MER and shows curiosity and motivation to helping and understanding, the mother may offer her case as an opportunity to the provider.

Chapter Eight
Life After D-MER

How each mother handles her D-MER is going to be different, as is how D-MER may or may not affect her after her breastfeeding journey has ended. It seems that especially for the milder experiences of D-MER that once it corrects, either through time or through weaning, D-MER becomes an increasingly distant recollection as time goes on. However, every mother and her post-D-MER experience can be just as different. There are mothers who experienced a tragic life event while dealing with D-MER and the two are still associated and tied together in their minds. Mothers who dealt with D-MER as well as other mental health issues may also feel that they had more of a self-altering experience while they breastfed. Some mothers have chosen to change how many children they wanted to have because nursing through D-MER again was nearly an inevitable part of growing in family size, and it was not worth the cost of experiencing it again. A small number of mothers have also reported having occasional D-MER-like experiences long after D-MER had stopped being an issue and long after they stopped lactating. A mother's time dealing with her D-MER, in the present, is going to affect and impact each mother differently in the future, some not at all and some more significantly. The following are some examples, that are neither all inclusive nor are they in the majority of outcomes.

Cognitive Effects

D-MER can bring along a new level of emotional regulation, intelligence, cognitive processes or awareness. Living day to day with a roller coaster of emotional changes that occur because of D-MER, as normal existence, creates an enormous emotional work load for a mother. It is impossible to cover all the possible variances that may occur in a mother's cognitive and emotional function due to this, and many would report no changes to their overall relationship with themselves once D-MER is behind them. However, there are some things that have occurred for a proportion of women, and they encounter and report some lasting psychological effects from this physiological problem. As one mother recounted, *"this experience of dealing with D-MER for over a year had a very negative and deep impact on me. Six months after weaning I still feel that I went through a very strange form of psychological torture, as I was forced, in a way, to experience extremely unpleasant feelings every few hours, every single day for over a year. I would sometimes hide in a different room and cry for a few minutes before having to breastfeed my hungry baby because I was dreading what was about to happen. I also felt all alone dealing with this problem as the one doctor I spoke to about this had never heard of such a thing, and I found myself amid an extremely pro-breastfeeding culture and unable to talk with anyone about the possibility of stopping breastfeeding early (which I now understand I obviously should have done). I am angry and hurt when I think about this experience, especially feeling so trapped and disempowered to do anything about it. I have trouble seeing women breastfeeding, or seeing pictures or advertisements of this, because I am reminded of what that awful sensation felt like. I can not bear to have my husband (or child accidentally) touch my nipples in any way. I now wear a bra 24 hours a day even while sleeping because I do not want to risk anything accidentally brushing up against that area and triggering the memories."* It is possible that for some mothers their experience with D-MER may influence their relationship with themselves in a way that may be more negative than positive. This kind of effect would be more likely for a mother with severe D-MER, and for a mother who is dealing with D-MER while at the same time struggling with mood disorders or life stressors. D-MER is likely to make additional life stressors harder for a mother to make sense of her experiences and work through them. Some mothers may find that they are still struggling with feelings of self shame or anxiety even once D-MER itself is no longer an issue. A mother related, *"post-breastfeeding my last child, I believe anxiety issues came to the forefront after*

D-MER. *Many times in my life I had been able to push away anxiety so that it was manageable. I have no idea what role dopamine plays in all of this, but post-breastfeeding, post-kids, I feel like I have lost some ability to "push through" anxiety.*" In such cases it is very possible that Cognitive Behavioral Therapy (CBT) with a therapist could be instrumental in helping the mother to gain greater understanding of herself and her emotional life. Additionally, CBT may equip her with new skills for coping with her feelings as she moves out of her experience with D-MER.

Perfectionism

The feelings experienced during D-MER are often so self directed that a mother may try to avoid saying or doing things that she may internally question or experience self-disgust about during an episode of D-MER. In response to this, perfectionism, which initially served as a self-protective strategy, can become a more permanent feature in a mother's life, even when she no longer experiences D-MER. One mother divulged how she was affected by this line of thinking, *"D-MER really made me become so self vigilant. It was exhausting. For example, perhaps my daughter gets her feelings hurt at the playgroup and I deal with that, move on, and then go to nurse my baby. My D-MER may feel more like hopelessness and sadness as I try to sort out the feelings. Sure, the emotions are not "real"... it's not because of the playground incident, it's because of the D-MER. But when I spontaneously try to connect it to something, that's what fits. Maybe later my husband calls and tells me that the checkbook bounced. I accept this news and go on with life, but when I nurse my baby I experience*

D-MER and it feels more like anxiety, but anxiety over the news my husband delivered to me. Later, someone at the grocery store criticizes me for wearing my baby, I go home and nurse her and my D-MER is suddenly construed as irritation or embarrassment, directly projected onto the grocery store event. So, I personally feel like everything in my life has to be perfect, so that there are not any other emotions to cause me to think that it's anything more than just D-MER, and then I can really say to myself "this is not real." Easy enough right? Have an uncomplicated stress free life and you can know when your D-MER hits, nothing is really wrong!" This mother found herself in a constant place of projecting her D-MER onto day to day events, which is not uncommon. When there is an emotional reaction, it is natural to look for the source. Mothers with D-MER are in a position of trying to go against this biological instinct and write off their emotional discomfort as nothing to worry about. This is something that is not easily done, and consciously or subconsciously trying to combat that with perfectionism is a rational response. Admittedly, it is impossible and can be very limiting to take this turn in cognitive functioning, but it is one way that D-MER can affect and shape a mother.

Echo Dysphoria

Some mothers report lingering emotional experiences, coined echo dysphoria, that are very familiar to D-MER, after they have finished nursing. The experience is not much different from the fact that mothers often report that the sensation of D-MER is ghostly familiar to them; a feeling they vaguely recognize, but cannot truly place. After having D-MER it is not surprising that even when mothers are done nursing, there may be other times in their lives that they experience something similar. D-MER is something so sudden and intense that after experiencing if for many months, a similar feeling is then going to be distinctly linked to D-MER. So in this case, now instead of being more like an unplaceable ghost dysphoria, it is a recognizable echo dysphoria, easily connected back to all those times of breastfeeding. One mother said, *"I am 48 years old and discovering this "disorder" has brought me relief from my life-long battle with D-MER. Yes, I said life long. Although I did feel moderate to severe D-MER while nursing all four of my children, I recognized that "yucky feeling" immediately after I nursed my first-born 28 years ago. I distinctly remember lying in bed as a child, waking up in the middle of the night and getting this yucky feeling that was always accompanied with an intense thirst. Since I was only about four or five, I thought it was just a very nasty way to experience thirst and called my mother for a drink of water. I have not breastfed for fourteen years, yet, I still can get that wave of yuckiness along with that let down feeling in my breasts (without the milk ejection) if I am in very uncomfortable situations. What's up with that?! Why do I still have this?! Am I the only one that has always felt this?! Help!"*. Whether echo dysphoria is another hormonal conglomeration, similar to what a D-MER mother has, or an emotional experience in response to a life experience, it is hard to say.

New Emotional Awareness And Intelligence
On a more positive note, most mothers who have shared their long-term effects of D-MER had good things to express. Some observed that they were more in tune with themselves

148

emotionally and otherwise. A mother stated, *"after D-MER I am more aware how emotion and thought is influenced by physiological processes so when I'm feeling low, I look at my physical health to help deal with the emotional side too"*. Mothers with D-MER are often faced with the reality that emotions are something that they cannot control, that D-MER or not, emotions have a physiological and biological role and cause in the human life. Some mothers are able to get better understanding of the difference between the uncontrollable emotional reactions that humans experience and the tangible response that can be chosen as a result. For mothers with D-MER, the response chosen in face of the reaction is dismissal of the experience because it is happening because of letdown, not because they are being threatened in any way.

Concerns About Future Breastfeeding Experiences

It is hard to tell a mother who is looking forward to nursing a new baby that she will in all likelihood be faced with D-MER again. There have been only a handful of reported instances when this was not the case for a mother who had a subsequent child after having D-MER with a previous one. For the majority of mothers, it will be something that she needs to be prepared for and expect. Hopefully in time, there will be easily accessed treatment options for mothers who choose to take that route. Having the knowledge and understanding of what D-MER is makes it a more bearable experience for many mothers, and breastfeeding a new baby far outweighs the negatives of going through D-MER again. But this does not alter the fact that there are mothers that are choosing formula feeding or altering family size in order to avoid the discomfort of D-MER. One mother accounted, *"I did not have D-MER with my first son but I did have it with my second son. It solidified my decision to only have two children.*" The near certain reoccurrence of D-MER with future children is a hard and regrettable place for a mother to be when her hopes are set on being able to comfortably breastfeed additional children. Another mother articulated, *"I am incredibly glad I finally finished breastfeeding and thankful I do not have to go through that right now. I am very afraid of experiencing D-MER again when my second child is born. I am already planning to formula feed at least partially from day one no matter what so I can easily switch completely if need be, but I am dreading having to go through the involuntary letdowns in the beginning even if I decide to formula feed exclusively."* The impact of D-MER in this way can be far reaching and change a mother's previous choices and goals.

Relief In Moving Forward

For a lot of mothers, D-MER is an isolated experience that they have, deal with and move on from peacefully. A mother accounted, *"I had a hard time explaining this feeling to the people in my life, especially because no one had heard of it. It brought up a lot of old feelings and emotions that I feel like I am still processing. I felt like I was going crazy because of the D-MER and every other person was able to push through their breastfeeding struggles. The funny thing is, as soon as I stopped breastfeeding my relationship with my kids improved immediately. I felt more confident and attached to them as soon as the physical effects stopped. I became so much more relaxed and fun again...the mom I pictured myself to be. Living up to other people's expectations of me was really intertwined with all of this,*

and contributed to the emotional toll D-MER took on me."
For most mothers, even those with severe D-MER, they are
able to look back on their time nursing through D-MER with
no regrets and no negative effects. But there is always relief
when D-MER is no longer part of a mother's life, whether
through self-correction or the baby having weaned. Though
the day to day toll that D-MER takes on a mother is intense,
in retrospect it often becomes just a thing that happened and
that the mother went through with her child. In the next
chapter are some stories from mothers who have written
about their journeys through D-MER.

Chapter Nine
Mother's Stories

Some mothers from the Facebook D-MER page were
gracious enough to provide their stories about their
experience with D-MER. Each one is unique as they faced
different types of challenges and had various outcomes with
how they managed and dealt with their D-MER. The essays
are included here as a way of helping a mother with D-MER
recognize that, though her experience has individual
elements, that her struggle is similar to others and that she is
not alone.

By Bonnie:

I always expected to get postpartum depression. I planned
for it. I knew the warning signs. With my history of regular
depression, I was sure the birth of my child would exacerbate
my long standing mental health issues.

As such, I was not surprised to find myself sitting in utter despair; feeling like the world was crashing down around me, clutching my wailing newborn to my breast just a few short days after arriving home from the hospital. I felt horrible, like my throat had dropped to the pit of my stomach. I was desperately thirsty, yet could not keep the water from leaking out of my eyes and down my face. There was a crushing sense of impending doom, though I had no idea what it was that I was afraid of. But I knew I needed help.

Fast forward fifteen minutes. My snuggled up baby was delightfully "milk drunk", and my loving husband and I lay on the floor beside her, marveling at her tiny perfect fingers, lips, everything. I could smell the turkey soup my mother was making in my kitchen, and I smiled. Being a new parent was exhausting, but wonderful. I would not trade it for anything.

I expected to get postpartum depression. I planned for it. I knew the warning signs. At least, I thought I did. But somehow, all of my preparation had not prepared me for what I was experiencing. Ninety five percent of my day was a picture perfect "new parent" experience, filled with sleepy baby snuggles and lots of baby poop. The other five percent of my day was pure hell, and it usually happened when I was breastfeeding.

My husband was also keeping a watchful eye out for postpartum depression, and would ask how I was doing. Most of the time, my answer was "exhausted but great". If he tried to talk to me while I was nursing the baby, my response was sharp, rude, and distracted. It was clear even to him that something about breastfeeding was not right.

The hospital where my daughter was born had provided a lactation consultant while we were there. Being a very private person, the idea of another woman looking at my swollen breasts and talking about my nipples made me very uncomfortable. I spent as little time with her as I could get away with, and I sure was not going to call her for help after I got home.

"Call your doctor", my husband urged. "And talk about how I cry when my baby nurses? She will just think I'm depressed, but I really do not think I am," I replied.

"What about the psychiatrist?" My husband suggested. "I'm certainly not going to talk about women boob problems to him!" I snapped.

Days, maybe weeks, went by. Finally, after a particularly horrible nursing session late one night, I turned to Google for answers. "Feeling horrible while breastfeeding" was my first Google search, and I half expected to find nothing. But instead, right in front of me, I found evidence that my experience was not unique. Here were stories of other women who described how I felt. There was a whole website describing the condition, and providing a physiological explanation for the whole thing. I was not crazy, and I was not depressed.

The relief of knowing was immense. I read everything Google could find me on this condition, called D-MER. As I read, I wondered: Why had no one warned me about this? If this was really a thing, why did not the hospital tell me about it?

Just knowing there was an explanation for how I felt, and possible strategies that might help was so freeing. I felt free to disregard the exaggerated emotions I felt. I felt free to stop worrying that I secretly hated my baby. I felt free to ask not to be disturbed, even by my husband, while I nursed. I felt free to continue breastfeeding my baby for as long as I chose to.

By Chloe:

I would be my happy self, enjoying my baby and feeling like the luckiest girl alive. That is, until I had to feed him. I would sit with my eyes shut while my letdown happened and the dark, homesick feeling would crash over me like I wave. I genuinely believed it was happening because I did not love my baby and could not bear him to be near me. But I could not understand why I felt that only when I fed him. Surely, I should feel nothing but joy and pride while my baby drank this amazing substance I had produced from my breasts?

After about four long months of suffering will this horrible feeling, my mother and I decided I must go to the doctor and see if anything could be done.

Approaching the doctor I felt ashamed and embarrassed. I was afraid she might think I did not love my new baby; that she could think it's because I was only nineteen and was struggling with becoming a parent. What if she even considered involving the social services? As I sat and

154

explained the dreadful feeling that took me every time I fed for around thirty to forty seconds, she nodded and labeled me as suffering from postnatal depression. I was so relieved that I finally had a label for the feeling, and that there was medication for it.

Weeks went on after I started my new medication that treated depression, and nothing had changed. That poisonous feeling was still at the pit of my stomach, swallowing me up with every feed. I decided to go back to the doctors, thinking she must have given me the wrong medication, and that must be why it had not fixed me. When I told the doctor this time that I was still having those feelings five, six, seven, times a day, she was confused and told me to stay on the medication, and that it should fix me soon.

I felt like a failure and that no one could ever fix me. I felt as though I needed to just admit to myself that I did not have a bond with my baby. I seriously considered just weaning him onto bottles and keeping him at arm's length. But what stopped me was when I was not feeding or having a letdown, I loved my baby more than life itself. So I bore through it all alone. Alone, except still with this nasty monster waiting in the pit of my stomach to pounce when I fed my beautiful young baby.

One morning I was happier than usual, ready to have a great day with my partner and our bundle of joy, until I had to feed my baby before we left. When that wave hit me, I finally decided to Google 'feeling sad when breastfeeding' and see if anyone suffered with it too. As soon as I saw that other ladies had written about that lingering feeling of guilt and despair, a wave of relief came over me and I could not help but cry. I still do not know if they were happy tears from knowing that someone knew how I felt, or whether it was because this 'thing' had a label, D-MER. I felt so much better knowing that it had a label. Though I did wonder, why did my doctor not know this? Why did they not diagnose me?

The following week I decided to go to a breastfeeding support group and speak to a health visitor about my condition. When I did, she was shocked and actually disgusted. She had never heard of this condition and told me she was sure it did not exist. Enraged, I told her I was living proof that it exists and I'd lived with this demon condition since the day my baby was born. It had made me feel alone, deranged and unfit to be a mother. This condition nearly stopped me from doing what I had loved doing for my baby, giving him my home made ingredients for life. I told the health visitor how D-MER made me feel. I showed her the D-MER website and how relieved I was that my condition had a label, that I could tell myself it was just a physiological response, and that I was not a bad mother, and that I loved my baby.

My hope is that all health professionals that are supposed to have the knowledge to support us breastfeeding mothers come to learn about this condition, and to understand it. I hope that D-MER is talked about, and that mothers know where to turn, without feeling like a liar or a freak. I hope that they do not suffer alone, behind closed doors, worrying about being judged and incorrectly labeled.

By Jacqueline:

When people hear that I've never had any nipple pain, latch issues, or supply issues, their first reaction is to exclaim how lucky I am...But they have no idea that I would trade just about anything to have those problems instead of this condition.

At first I thought my D-MER symptoms were psychological because of how nervous I was to breastfeed. Then I thought it was a conditioned response because my daughter would get very fussy after feeding (colic and reflux). As she got older and the fussiness subsided, I wondered when the negative feelings would go away. As the weeks and months went on, I slowly resigned myself to the possibility it would never go away, and that my body could not handle breastfeeding. I also feared that it meant I did not love my daughter and that I was not connecting with her. It's hard to convey the scope of devastation it causes.

One day, I read about D-MER in "The Womanly Art of Breastfeeding". I could not believe it! What I was going through had a name! I was not crazy. I immediately told my husband about it and joined the support groups on Facebook. Although it provided some much needed validation, it's very frustrating that there are no real answers. One of the most difficult aspects of D-MER is the lack of awareness and understanding of its impact. No one I've told has ever heard of it. My doctor's look at me with confused faces, and loved ones can be a bit dismissive because they do not know much about it (Side note, my husband is very supportive, as he has witnessed first- hand what happens to

157

me when I let down). I feel betrayed by my body, robbed of what's supposed to be a joyous experience, and am still grieving what could have been. I want to breastfeed for a year, and I'm 7 months in. It has been one of the most difficult experiences of my life, and I cannot stress enough my yearning for answers and a treatment. Despite all of this, I'm so thankful that my body is able to provide the nourishment my daughter needs, and I'm proud that I've made it this far.

By Margaret:

My experience with D-MER went so smoothly, I can hardly take credit for finding something that helped. Relief found me.

When I gave birth to my third child, I already had a four year old and two year old at home. We had just bought our first house, and baby number three was born less than a week before Christmas. My life felt like a whirlwind. My older two children seemed to be fighting all the time. I'd sigh as I sat down to nurse their little brother and just feel exasperated, anxious, with butterflies in my stomach. I assumed these feelings stemmed from life changes and being exhausted from little sleep.

Around six or seven weeks postpartum, however, I began to notice that this odd feeling in the pit of my stomach did not just happen when the older two were fighting, or because I was feeling overwhelmed with parenting three littles, or from still not being fully unpacked from moving. It did, however, happen just about every time I started nursing. Guzzling water for the first minute or so provided some relief from the anxious feelings. Even if I did not drink water, I noticed that the feeling faded away after a minute or two. I held on to that fact every time I sat to nurse the baby.

The symptoms were not powerful, but they began to puzzle me. I had not experienced it with my first two. So, at my son's eight week check-up, I asked his pediatrician if she had ever heard of such symptoms. She had not, but explained it was likely something physiological happening when my milk letdown. She did not have a remedy, but I left with the happy reassurance that I probably was not crazy. I went home and scoured the internet. Success! A single website, devoted to these odd symptoms associated with letdown. I definitely was not crazy! And I was not alone!

The next day, life went on a little easier. I knew what this thing called D-MER was, that I had it, and that I was fortunate to have a very mild case of it. I visited my chiropractor that day, saying nothing to her about D-MER and having no clue that this visit would be pivotal in my D-MER story. After talking about general health concerns, I left her office with a bottle of vitamin D drops. She recommended I take fourteen drops (7000 i/u) daily— enough to benefit me and my breastfed child.)

Fast forward two weeks. I was nursing the baby in our quiet house when suddenly, it hit me! There were not any butterflies when I started to nurse him. In fact, I could not even pinpoint the last time I had D-MER symptoms. I was shocked! From what I had read, D-MER did not seem to be something that went away all that quickly. What had changed? Vitamin D drops. I scoured the internet. I already knew that D-MER was most likely related to an intense drop in dopamine levels at the time of letdown. Okay, Google... Dopamine and vitamin D. Wait, what? Vitamin D activates the body's release of dopamine! I'm not a doctor or scientist, but it sure seemed obvious to me that vitamin D was my relief from D-MER.

I continued to take my fourteen drops of vitamin D daily until the bottle was empty. Symptom-free for weeks, I decided to try going without the drops to see if I was completely cured. After several days, I noticed occasional twinges of the butterflies at letdown. So, I purchased more vitamin D and continued taking it for the next few months. At the time I am writing this, my son is thirteen months old and I still nurse him a couple of times each day. I have a bottle of vitamin D on top of my refrigerator, but most days I forget to take any. I do not remember the last time I had any D-MER symptoms, but I will never forget what it felt like: exasperated, anxious, and butterflies in my stomach. Not everyone's D-MER story has as happy of an ending—not everyone will find relief so easily, but I hope my story helps at least a few women through their D-MER journey.

By Autumn:

I guess the beginning of my story is deciding to breastfeed in the first place. My partner was very encouraging and adamant that I at least try to breastfeed. I was willing, but always said I would bottle feed when necessary without hesitation. I have a son as well as the daughter I was about to welcome, and I had never attempted to breastfeed him. I suffered a controlled but grievous postpartum depression after my son was born, and was hoping that this time around I could avoid that. As my son wanted, I could feed continuously because breastmilk Is digested so efficiently, and with some luck, I could also get some sleep! So began the journey. About eight hours, after an induced labor, I welcomed my sweet girl. Within five minutes she latched on, and quite literally, now at almost two years old, has been attached to me since! But that first latch and those after began to feel strange to me.

I rationalized that I had just given birth. I was raw and emotional. And so happy! Happier than I had ever been, truly. My daughter was all I had dreamed of and more; I was not exhausted, but rejuvenated! But, as time settled into twenty-four hours postpartum, I could not shake the odd feeling I had every time she latched on. I would be beyond thrilled to hear that little squeak beside my hospital bed, coming from my swaddled newborn, ready to be with me. I would lay awake, when I should have been resting and long for her to need me. I would bring her to my chest and she would settle in, and then, as if slowly plummeting in a dream to my inevitable death, I would sink into a fog that felt like I had been drugged. I was not in the room. My fiancé could sense a change in me from across the room. The second the clouds descended on me, I was changed. My mood was different. I was sad, and thirsty, and needing of something. I felt like I could never be enough for this precious child I had been given. And then, I would feel calm once more, and capable, as if the past few minutes did not happen. I would hold my baby, burp her, change her, and nurse her some more. And mostly while in the hospital, my symptoms were not completely unpleasant...some times when my milk would let down, I would be deliriously happy; but almost too happy, a little hysterical, even. And so, I began to mention to my nurses and consultants that I felt strange when my daughter latched on. Every single person I said this to suggested PPD. But this was not PPD. I was beyond happy and felt ready to take care of my family...except, that pesky latch. What was going on?

Once we were home and settled in, I continued to experience the bouts of mood shifts while we breastfed. They did not last long and, for me at least, were manageable; but I was still curious as to what was happening, and lived in a bit of limbo, fearing that at any moment I would spiral into full blown depression. But I never did; my daughter was thriving and I did not mind feeding her. She slept well, and I myself was relatively rested. But by then I knew that when I needed to breastfeed, I had better brace myself for the inevitable surge of negative emotion that would at times flash all of my greatest fears straight before my eyes. I became frightened not knowing whether I would have a mild episode or if I would have guilt ridden, tormented let down? It was rough for awhile.

But then one day, while browsing my social media, I came across a post about D-MER. I was in a lot of mommy groups online, and breastfeeding support was pretty much all I was reading at the time. All at once, D-MER became manageable for me. It finally had a name, I finally had a name, and what I was experiencing did not mean that I was losing my sanity along with my heart to my daughter. I was going to be ok, because this was real! And while I say D-MER became manageable, it was by an odd turn. Through soaking up information online, I learned that distraction is the key to fighting the negative symptoms of D-MER. I mostly distracted myself by learning as much as possible about this rarely spoken of condition. It helped me to get through the falls by understanding that my body was adjusting for the needs of my child; and that if I just rode it out; I would be longingly looking at my sweet child again soon enough.

Sometimes, D-MER can present as feeling incredibly "touched out" and this has been worse for me as my daughter has grown. She will be two next month and we are at the end of our breastfeeding journey. Although I have breastfed for an honorable amount of time, and I feel like I've given her beyond enough of the benefit from breastfeeding, I still ultimately feel like D-MER played a role in the way we quit. My moods had begun to get touchy again after a year and a half of very satisfying breast only feeding. I started to feel annoyed that she wanted to suck at me and hold on, squeezing my breasts and groping and being a two year old ;and she suddenly did not seem as satisfied with feeds. I got to where I felt the "yuck" feeling of D-MER again, but through entire feed. It was time to stop in every way.

When I look to the future, I cannot help but wonder what menopause will be for me. I've read that D-MER sufferers can have similar symptoms again when they experience menopause. We shall see, I suppose. For now, I would like to help in any way to help others understand their body and what changes occur after birth. That is my wish.

By Marianna:

Throughout my pregnancy I dealt with depression off and on. I had discussed this with my OBGYN, who referred me to a counselor so that I would have support during and after pregnancy. A few weeks after giving birth to my first child on Sept 25th, 2016, I began to recognize the negative emotions I was flooded with before "milk let down" as D-MER. I became aware of D-MER through a Breastfeeding Support group on Facebook. Had I not seen a post by another mother suffering, I may have never known what was wrong. I began to research and tried to build the confidence to talk to my doctor.

My first attempt to reach out about my struggle with D-MER was to my counselor. I'm not sure why I thought she would have any idea what I was talking about, but I was suffering and desperate for support. I tried to explain the condition and her first question was, "What is a let down?" I felt more isolated, more alone, and more helpless. A few weeks later I spoke with my primary care physician through blurry eyes, who nodded understandingly and said she had not heard of D-MER but went on to say "it makes sense, since hormones are all out of whack from pregnancy." That was the extent of the conversation. Finally I built up the courage to attend a Breastfeeding Support Group at my local hospital. I checked in and sat down to nurse my now four month-old daughter. A lactation consultant came over to ask how I was doing. I began to express that I was battling something called D-MER. She asked if I was trying to say "that I have a strong let down." I shook my head and she could tell there was

164

something more going on. She asked me to wait a minute while she spoke with the other lactation consultant. Moments later a consultant with a warm spirit approached me and began to express her sympathy. She knew exactly what D-MER was and showed compassion towards me. She told me in her twenty years as a lactation consultant, she had only seen three other patients who suffered from D-MER, and I was given a printed handout with information and tips. Before I left that day she caught me and said, "I know it must be hard to come out and nurse in public. I just want you to know you're doing a great job." That was the first time I really felt like someone knew what I was going through, and actually cared. I never knew that what I needed to get through D-MER was sympathy: knowing that someone cared, and that someone was proud of me for sticking it out.

By Cassie:

I'm hesitant to share my story here because I was not sure I was going to make it breastfeeding long enough to make me feel as though my story was significant. So many mommas with D-MER have made it months and years into their breastfeeding journey, and I'm honestly jealous!

I realized over several weeks that I needed to make a different choice if I was going to look back on my son's first year with happy memories. I dealt with depression as a teenager, and it took me eight years to get though it and manage my own mental/emotional health naturally and without medication. It's been five years since I felt like my life was not in my control. Fast forward to the present---My son is now ten weeks old.

The first few days of breastfeeding were wonderful. Even though we had trouble latching, he adjusted fine to using the nipple shield and I was able to pump colostrum for him in the hospital. I felt the warm fuzzies and was amazed at how much I loved breastfeeding. Weeks two through four were marked by sadness though. Every time I sat down to feed or pump I would cry. I chalked it up to my hormones still being out of whack, yet he still struggled to latch so we would nurse half the time, and the rest I just pumped for him. I could pump forty eight ounces a day! Around week six I started searching for information to explain why I still cried, got these terrible thoughts and just basically felt horrible about myself every time I let down. It was like running a mental marathon every time I pumped.

That's when I found out about D-MER. I found comfort in knowing I was not nuts and it made some feedings/pumps easier. I decided to stop nursing regularly and only pump every six hours. That way I only had to work through those feelings four times a day. I still nursed my son if he or I needed the comfort from it. My lactation consultant was amazing, but did not know much about D-MER. The seventh week was the worst. It seemed like I spent entire days crying. I would have symptoms so bad all throughout my pumps and it would take hours afterwards to feel normal again. I was dealing with crippling guilt because all I wanted to do was stop breastfeeding. But how could I possibly justify stopping when I was able to produce forty or more ounces a day for my baby? How could I deny him that gift? I would stew in this all day long.

Since that week, I became been more proactive about my daily mental health, having good and bad days; and I just made the choice each morning to keep going. I then started supplementing with formula one feeding per day. He took that first formula bottle without any fuss or reaction--it might as well have been breast milk! I then dropped my pumps to three a day and made just enough for his daily intake if I supplement one feeding. My first goal that I set for myself when it started to get hard was that I wanted to make it long enough for him to get his first vaccines. That day came, and I was so proud that I had come that far; but honestly I was ready to be done with it. Every single day seemed like it lasted an eternity, and I felt like I missed out on joyful moments while I was trapped in the D-MER fog or the dread knowing I had to pump soon. I wanted to stop breastfeeding, but was afraid that I would get stuck in the same mom guilt that I had worked so hard to get through the past few weeks.

After that I ended up pumping twice a day until week thirteen, and then I just stopped. It took about two weeks for my milk to "dry up". I'm twenty weeks postpartum now and I've noticed that I still leak a drop here and there--like when showering or inspecting my now deflated and saggy new knockers. I thought for sure I would feel "back to normal" a few weeks after weaning, but instead I could not shake the fog that I was in. In hindsight, I think the fog was always there, but the hormone wave from my letdown intensified it greatly. It took me about a week to work up the nerve to call my doctor and talk about the lingering depression and anxiety I was experiencing. I've been on Bupropion SR twice a day for three weeks now and I'm feeling a lot better. I would not say that I am one hundred percent there, but definitely on my way. For the first time since my baby was born, I am experiencing feelings with him that I had almost forgotten about. The little bursts of joy and feelings of gratitude are returning as I become more present in the moments of my day. I feel like the first four months of his life were such a blur from the constant mental and emotional battles I was fighting inside. It feels like a lifetime has passed at the same time.

By Jessica:

I had D-MER with my first son but did not know that's what the dreadful feeling was. I assumed it was postpartum depression and was put on antidepressants. They did not help, but I understand why now. When my second son was a week old I Googled "bad feelings with letdown" and was immediately directed to the D-MER website. It was such a huge relief to know there was a medical reason for the way I was feeling. Unfortunately, the feeling of dread and despair was so intense that I weaned him at two weeks old. I was so relieved though, because I was able to formula feed him happily and bond with him without the pressure of breastfeeding and trying to stave off the dread.

When I was pregnant with my third son, I knew that I would likely have the symptoms of D-MER again and so my midwife and I decided we would try encapsulating my placenta to see if that would help. I made it to four months of breastfeeding with him, but the placenta pills did not seem to help at all and I was having major issues with oversupply and forceful letdown that was made worse by the anxiety of knowing I would be having the depressing symptoms of D-MER every time I had a letdown (which was about every thirty minutes because of the oversupply!)

When I was pregnant with my fourth child, I started taking a multitude of supplements during pregnancy that I was hoping would help with what I knew was coming. The midwife I saw during this pregnancy was willing to do some blood work and we identified several vitamins I was deficient in. Fortunately, by the time my daughter was born, I was at mostly normal levels and also started taking Rhodiola tincture. The tincture was the most effective at preventing the D-MER symptoms. I believe that since it helps with dopamine, and I have a history of having dopamine imbalances (depression and anxiety since my teen years), which is why it is so effective at helping. My midwife also worked diligently with me to make sure my supply was just right and that my daughter's tongue tie was revised so that breastfeeding was easier for both of us in every way.

My daughter is now twenty-two months old and still nursing. There are days that the D-MER is worse, and I know that I need to take better care of myself and work on my dopamine problems by increasing my supplements and outdoor time. However at this time, the D-MER symptoms are barely present most of the time, and I do not think of it very often at all.

By Manda:

I have been experiencing D-MER for nearly five years. I have breastfed two children through it, including three months of tandem feeding. D-MER is the reason I did not tandem feed for longer and had to wean my oldest child off the breast.

Breastfeeding is something I am incredibly passionate about. Both professionally (I am a midwife) and personally; I always knew breastfeeding was the only option for me. Artificially feeding was never an option, even after experiencing severe D-MER.

When I first started breastfeeding my oldest daughter nearly five years ago, I would experience a truly horrible feeling. It felt as if my soul, my life force, was being drained from my body. I was an empty shell. I was flat, unmotivated to do anything, uninterested in anything, and even breathing was a chore and a challenge. I was a husk of nothing. This tiny person was draining the life out of me. But then after about a minute, color would return to my world, I was resuscitated and my life returned. This would happen multiple times throughout a feed in varying degrees. Every time letdown would occur, I died a little bit inside. At first, I thought it was normal. I thought it was part of me realizing what my life involved as a new mum. Not once did I ever think of quitting breastfeeding, despite the fact that this feeling never went away. It faded and was less intense as the months and years went on, but was always there, every single feed.

When my oldest daughter was two and a half, my youngest daughter was born. Once again, breastfeeding was my only option and I just did it. I was also still breastfeeding my oldest, although I had encouraged her to limit it to one a day. I tandem fed my girls for three months. In those three months, I never thought the D-MER could be stronger than it was when I first started breastfeeding. I was wrong. Not only was I an empty shell when feeding, that shell began to crack. I began to fall apart in ways I did not even know possible. Suicidal thoughts made their way into what was left of me numerous times. But all this always only lasted for about a minute, and I would soon be back to normal.

After three months, I could not do it anymore. The thought of breastfeeding was terrifying. I was so afraid and anxious at the thought of going back into that black hole every time I would sit down to feed. The thought of just not doing it ever again crossed my mind, but that would mean my three month-old would not get fed. The day the thought of starving my daughter was more appealing than breastfeeding her, I knew something needed to change, and needed to change immediately.

I then weaned my oldest, and it was painfully forced. She went cold turkey with no reason she could understand and no input into the matter. It was horrible and painful and there were tears from all of us. But it was better than the alternative. She still asked for 'milkies' daily for the next year. I still experienced the D-MER, but my shell did not crack anymore. I was back to the empty husk of nothing only. And I could handle that, because I knew I had handled it before.
I am still breastfeeding my youngest, and over two years later the D-MER has faded, but never gone away. I still get it

occasionally if I am extra tired, or stressed or hungry. But I take it. I hold on tight and ride the ride, because I know it will not last forever.

I am so glad that despite it I was able to still have that special experience with my girls. The breastfeeding relationship is something I can never get back. And for me as a mum, I know I put my girls first, and I always will.

By Marianne:

I was lucky: I found out what D-MER was. That is, at least, the second time around. The first time I was not able to keep up feeding past the first few weeks, so D-MER may well have been mixed in amongst the general anxiety I had at that time.

The second time round though, I was more prepared; I'd successfully bottle-fed and weaned my then almost three year old. I started off by combination feeding and, despite continued pain and other medical issues, my son and I started to get the knack of exclusive breastfeeding. New to the breastfeeding world I searched around for reliable and not too didactic information about how to make it a success. Thankfully I happened upon the Kelly Mom website which had all sorts of useful, well researched information – including an article titled 'Depression or other negative emotions upon milk letdown (D-MER)'. This rang a few bells with me. Even whilst pregnant I was aware of sudden low feeling sweeping across me. But I'd suffered with ante-natal depression and anxiety in both pregnancies, and assumed it was all part and parcel of the same problem. However, since

172

giving birth, my anxiety and depression had significantly improved – yet still these feelings remained.

Finding out that D-MER is an actual, diagnosable condition with a name that others suffer from it was the first step in being able to manage the condition, as was finding out that it's causes were physiological rather than psychological was step two. It was this that gave me the tools to 'get through' D-MER on a daily basis.

With my cloudy memories of that (very) sleepless year, I do not actually remember much about D-MER whilst feeding. Probably the fact I was feeding my baby or cuddling him whilst he slept, eighty percent of the time meant that it all melded together. It definitely happened, but my memories of D-MER whilst feeding are fuzzy. Although, I remember the spontaneous letdowns that occurred when I had those elusive moments to myself – in the shower or driving for example, and those memories are much clearer. In fact, I knew I would have a letdown and experience D-MER every time I had a shower and became prepared for it.

It would often take me a moment to realize what was happening - when those strangely nostalgic feelings of self-loathing and hopelessness crept up on me. Once I had come to expect it though it became easier to identify it happening. By a few months in I knew I had to grit my teeth and talk myself through to the other side 'everything is going to be ok', 'this is not real', 'deep breaths'. The times I really was alone I would shout, or grunt in the style of a tennis player, as a cathartic release – that really helped. Then I would wait for the letdown. The letdown would be my reassurance that I was right – my 'I told you so' to myself. The despair would try and trick me every time though – it felt so real. The letdown sensation felt like a shield, reminding me that what I'd read was true; D-MER does exist and is a physiological phenomenon instead of a psychological one.

However, I was always left with the fallout afterwards. When such negative feelings have consumed your brain, even only for a minute, it takes a while to shake them off. Whilst the feelings of despair lasted only thirty seconds or so, the sense of disappointment in myself lingered, and again I had to remind myself that it was all a trick, and in reality nothing was different from a few minutes before.

I fear if I had not discovered more about D-MER the ongoing persistence of negative thoughts could well have brought on a resurgence of the anxiety and depression I had suffered from in pregnancy. I am, therefore, forever grateful that I was able to find out more. I sincerely hope that D-MER will become more recognized by medical professionals and breast-feeding consultants in order to help others suffering from this condition in the future.

By Leianna:

Those first months of being a momma are a blur, so I do not remember the first time it happened. My first memory of what I later learned was D-MER was sitting on the couch next to my husband crying my eyes out as I nursed my son, who was only a few weeks old. I had no idea why I was crying, and my poor husband did not either. We both felt helpless, and I just remember him telling our dog, who was

174

leaning his furry head on my lap, "Good boy for comforting Momma."

For me, D-MER most often presented itself with uncontrollable sobbing. The middle-of-the-night feedings were usually the worst. I felt irritated, anxious, and panicky-- like there was no way I could keep doing this. I was never diagnosed by a medical professional, but I also think some of my symptoms were more commonly attributed to breastfeeding aversion. However, I was not breastfeeding while pregnant, or breastfeeding an older child, which are the most common scenarios for breastfeeding aversion. Sometimes the physical feeling of breastfeeding just utterly disgusted me—in a panicky, intolerable way, and I had to suddenly unlatch my poor son, leaving us both sobbing. No matter what symptoms were happening, most times, I would try to 'power through' and sit there nearly hyperventilating, biting my hand, or kicking my legs to numb the other feelings I was having. Then, as quickly as it all started, I would feel fine and cheerful again-- an almost invigorating feeling of relief would come over me. Maybe I could keep breastfeeding for a few more days... maybe even weeks.

My mom visited when my son was about a month old, and helped me call lactation consultants for help, but D-MER was all new to them too. Our son's pediatrician had not heard of it. At my six week post-natal checkup, I asked my doctor (a male) about it, but he had never heard of such a thing either. He said weaning was an option, but that obviously my son would benefit from continuing breastfeeding; and since it was only happening about once a day, he did not think it was worth pursuing more diagnosis or treatment. He more or less recommended just "toughing it out." Bu that was easy for him to say.

By this point I had discovered D-MER.org, and at least knew I was not alone. I found out my sister-in-law had also gone through it, and we exchanged emails of our experiences -- that helped a little. I also eventually requested a home visit from a lactation consultant. She had only recently heard of D-MER, but came prepared with suggestions to help. (Most of which I had already found, since there are so few resources out there on the subject...)

Some of her suggestions were helpful though: I started a daily log of especially bad D-MER episodes, when I ate food was thought to be a trigger, and other factors such as lack of sleep and dehydration. It eventually helped me to see a little bit of a pattern, so I could at least understand why some days were worse, even if I was not very good at preventing it—getting enough sleep as a new mom? Yeah, right! I also started taking fish oil supplements to see if the extra DHA would help - and I believe it did.

Distraction, by watching TV shows on my tablet helped a little. My mom and I also discussed how, like with panic/anxiety attacks, you cannot talk yourself out of it... but you can talk yourself through it. It helped to remind myself that it would be over soon, and I would feel normal again in just a few minutes.

I was able to keep breastfeeding my son until he was almost eleven months old—with D-MER coming and going right up until the end. I had an abundant supply of breast milk from

176

the start—perhaps from incessant pumping while my son spent his first week of life in the NICU. Up until he was six months old, I was always pumping to add more to the freezer. I do not know if that extra supply increased my susceptibility to D-MER, but I am grateful to still be able to supplement my son's whole milk with breast milk even now at thirteen months.

My husband and I plan to have more children, and it already gives me anxiety thinking I will most likely have to go through D-MER again. But I survived it once, and I can do it again!

Chapter Ten
For Partners And Support People

For this section, the information is going to be presented as an open letter to those who support mothers who have dysphoric milk ejection reflex. The content is taken directly from mother's expressions of what they wish their support people knew about their struggles with D-MER. It holds the information and hidden feelings of vulnerable and frustrated mothers who want nothing more than to be supported and understood, in a way that is translatable to them.

Dear Partner,

Thank you for taking the time and for having the interest to read this. I value the fact that you want to understand my experience and I recognize that you strive to support me in the best way possible.

You know all those times where you have seen me struggling and you try to fix it but somehow things get worse because I just want you to hear and support me? This is pretty much another one of those times. I love the fact that you care for me so much that you want to fix anything that is bothering me, But in this case, the best way to "fix it" is by offering me your acceptance and support.

I know you won't be able to entirely understand how D-MER feels, and I know how hard it must be for you to see me struggle and to not be able to relate to my experience. But that is okay, I accept that. There are still a lot of ways you can help me feel better.

D-MER isn't a psychological issue but it does have an emotional impact. However, I am not crazy or hormonal or irrational and it's not histrionics of any kind. D-MER is a brain chemical thing. The chemicals and neurotransmitters that control the functions of lactation are basically being unkindly quirky in my case. It's all pretty sciency but it's out of my control and it's not my fault. In short, it makes me feel like emotional crap every time my milk releases. Which is a lot. I have milk letting down so often! During feedings, in-between feedings, when my breasts are too full, and when I hear the baby waking up. So, when my brain sends the message to my body to release the milk, dopamine is doing it's job wrong and I get this super negative emotional wave course through my whole body.

178

Yeah. Dopamine. Who knew? Apparently it is totally involved in the lactation process because prolactin can't help my body make the milk unless dopamine lowers a little to let prolactin levels rise. In science dopamine is called prolactin's "gate-keeper" because they have a very intwined relationship. You hear all over the place about how good dopamine can make us feel when levels go up and the opposite is true with low levels. My dopamine gets out of prolactin's way when I letdown, but it is dropping too fast or too low or something (science doesn't know which yet), and it makes me feel like super crap.

The feelings are intense. It's like my whole world is suddenly wrong and I can't do or control anything to make it right again. It makes me doubt myself, I feel like a bad mom, a bad partner, and a bad person. Everything seems hopeless and dark and I feel worthless during the wave. But it is just a wave, it is actually pretty short lived. Super bad, but super short. Really intense and pretty frequent. It's not postpartum depression though, once the wave is over and the neurotransmitters right themselves again, I have perspective back and things are as they were before. It's pretty crazy making stuff and that's why I really appreciate your patience. It's hard to keep it together when it is so derailing and sudden.

Here are some things that other moms with D-MER want their partner to know about what is helpful and what is not. Every experience is different, so I would love to talk about these suggestions together so that you can know which ones are important and helpful to me, specifically.

- D-MER sucks! Please be patient during my momentary lapse of reason.
- Sometimes I may not be able to answer your questions until the attack is over, so please be patient with me.
- Please entertain our older child. He is sweet when he tries to cuddle me and our baby during a breastfeed, but I can't handle it, I just feel like I want to jump out of my skin. Your help with the other kids during breastfeeding is awesome.
- I would appreciate it if you offered me a glass of water when I sit down to breastfeed. Drinking cold water during D-MER helps and sometimes I don't have time to get one myself.
- When I talk about my D-MER I don't need solutions, I just need you to listen. I know what it is and how it affects me and that it will stop, I just really need to vent to you sometimes. Nod your head, actively listen, and offer empathy without suggestions.
- Please don't look at me differently when I share with you the horrible emotions I feel about myself and our child with each latch. Remind me that I am, indeed, a great mother and that I am doing an amazing job.
- Remember that I don't know why I'm crying, I am not sad for an explainable reason, I am not having a bad day, and you haven't done anything wrong. Just give me a few minutes for it to pass and I will be fine. Having to try to explain myself makes it all so much harder.
- After spending all day and evening with a cluster feeding baby, I am all touched out. Even lovingly putting your head on my shoulder makes me want to run away. It's not because of you, it is just a phase of my mothering journey right now. I would like to find other ways to give and receive love and support right now.

- Please just make sure I have water, a blanket, turn the television on to a show I enjoy, and if you're feeling really generous, you can wash the dishes. Your acts of care-taking really go a long way.
- Please offer to take the baby for 5 minutes while I get some space to breathe sometimes. It feels better when you offer to help that way. It can be hard to ask for what I want and need.
- I don't want to stop breastfeeding despite the challenges of D-MER. I know it sounds like I am complaining about breastfeeding and I understand that your rational brain jumps to the conclusion of weaning. But my need to talk about my struggles doesn't mean I want to stop, it simply means I need more support in my journey.
- I can't explain my feelings, because I don't understand the experience myself. Just know that it is happening and it happens every time. Please don't ask every time that I nurse whether I'm feeling it again. I am.
- I need help, not advice. I need support, not judgment. I need love, not resentment.
- I'm not over-reacting or making it up. Sometimes it feels like you think I am making a big deal out of a little thing. But, it is real and it is awful every single time I feed our baby.
- I'm sorry for lashing out when my D-MER has gotten the best of me.
- I'm not a hypochondriac, D-MER is very real and it is understood inside the scope of the science of lactation. You can't see what the chemicals are doing in my brain, but that doesn't mean that it's not a problem.
- I'm sorry you have to stand by and watch me go through it. I have a lot of guilt over your suffering and mine.

- I do not have postpartum depression. I am sad only while nursing.
- I need your sympathy even if you don't fully understand D-MER yourself. Please offer words like, "I know this is hard for you", "you are so committed, I am really proud of you", "I am here to support you", "I can see you are struggling, I wish I could help more", "hang in there, you are doing great", "I am sad for your feelings, but I have your back the whole way", "I know this is unfair for you, but I want you to know that you are such an amazing mom", "I want you to know that you can ask for what you need from me", "let me know how I can best help", "you are really courageous and I admire you", "you are so strong", "it is going to be okay".

Thank you again for taking the time to read this. You are a great problem solver and a great partner and I know you must struggle with not being able to solve this problem. I appreciate your love and support through all of this. I crave validation for my experience with D-MER. Going through it isn't easy, but breastfeeding is important to me and I want to try to persevere through this struggle. Most importantly, feel welcome to be openly curious about my experience, even though I can't explain my emotions well, because they aren't founded in reality. It is not about the house, or work, or the kids or your parents. Though I have feelings about those too! But the D-MER feelings are like a reflex. Like your knee. You don't want to move your leg, but when your knee is bumped in the right place, it kicks anyway. Reflexes can't be fixed, solved, easily explained or understood. That's the feeling of D-MER. But I love to be heard and have a listening and understanding presence supporting me along the way. Thank you for being that person.

All my love,
The mother of this beautiful child

Chapter Eleven
What Is Next For D-MER

Research into D-MER presents a unique opportunity, not only for the increased understanding of D-MER itself, but also for further understanding the science of lactation and other dopamine related conditions and diagnoses. Because D-MER seems to have such a predictable reaction, with such a sudden disturbance and recovery, it could be possible to measure what kind of activity dopamine has at the time of dysphoria with a single-scan dynamic molecular imaging technique.[69] This technology could perhaps offer insights into the process of dopamine release during MER, and thus, bring better understanding to the mechanism of D-MER. Other answers that mothers are looking for, other than "what makes D-MER happen?" (looking for mechanism) include "why do I have D-MER?" (looking for what causes it), "who else has D-MER?" (looking for commonalities and frequency of occurrence), "what other factors are included in my D-MER?" (looking at criteria for diagnosis/future neurotransmitter issues/predisposition), and "how do I fix my D-MER?" (looking at treatment). When and if these questions will be answered is unknown as there is no neuroscientific research on D-MER being worked on at this

[69] Prog Brain Res. Author manuscript; available in PMC 2014 Jul 8. Imaging dopamine neurotransmission in live human brain. Rajendra D. Badgaiyan

time. For the last several years the spreading of information and awareness has been the main focus for D-MER and will remain such until D-MER becomes an area of interest of the neuroscientific community.

Better Understanding Of D-MER

There are many hormones and chemicals at play within lactation, and there is new information about all of those being discovered through research regularly about the surrounding mechanisms.

For example, within the past few years, after D-MER's initial investigation and preliminary conclusions, a further study was done about oxytocin. Once thought to be simply the bonding and feel good hormone, one study also proposed that it can also strengthen distressing memories and can increase fear and anxiety.[70] Though a paradoxical effect of oxytocin was first considered for D-MER, there was no evidence of this other side of oxytocin at the time. It is not likely that this demeanor of oxytocin is fully responsible for D-MER, because the study does not link oxytocin as the originator of negative feelings, but instead suggests that "the hormone actually strengthens social memory in the brain." In this case, it could be that the heightened levels of oxytocin while a mother nurses with D-MER, could result in reverberation past the D-MER event and could trigger further fear and anxiety in further breastfeeding sessions. This is simple speculation, but it is used as an example of how little is known and understood, as well as to emphasize

---

[70] Science Daily. 'Love hormone' is two-faced: Oxytocin strengthens bad memories and can increase fear and anxiety. 2013. Northwestern University

the fact that science still has so much to learn about the hormones and chemicals underlying emotional experiences.

A better understanding of D-MER, its mechanism and what causes it, would be valued and appreciated information for the field of lactation. Not only is it important to be able to offer evidence based education and solutions whenever possible, but it would also give mothers awareness and peace of mind about their experience, add support to help work against premature weaning, and provide possible diagnostic treatment methods for mothers that have severe and debilitating D-MER.

Understanding Other Conditions

The predictable nature of D-MER and the technology available for studying it offers a unique opportunity, because other conditions or disorders that dopamine is responsible for have a much less predictable response. For many conditions that are speculated to be dopamine related, there are beliefs within the medical community that dopamine plays a role, though what role exactly, remains unknown. This is far from a conclusive list, but some of the conditions suspected of inappropriate dopamine activity are included here. The understanding of these conditions could possibly be furthered though further research of D-MER.

Restless leg syndrome (RLS) is a condition that results in involuntary leg movement when asleep. The exact cause is unknown and still speculative but many theories and studies have pointed in the direction of inadequate dopamine playing a part, if not being the culprit.[71]

Premenstrual dysphoric disorder (PMDD) is a diagnosable mood disorder. It is thought to be hereditary, and there are speculations that estrogen is involved, but additionally at fault could be dopamine; with theories that depleted prefrontal cortical dopamine contributes to PMDD.[72]

Parkinson's is a disease in which the neurons that produce dopamine become impaired causing less and less dopamine available in the circuit of the substantia nigra and multiple brain regions, causing impaired movement and loss of muscle coordination.[73]

Attention deficit hyperactivity disorder (ADHD) is also thought to be, at least partially, a dopamine mediated condition.[74] Dopamine levels or the efficiency of dopamine receptors in the brain are thought to be at fault and medications used to treat ADHD modulate the levels of

----

[71] Restless Legs Syndrome Fact Sheet from NIH Neurological Institute

[72] MedScape. Spotlight on PMDD: Hereditary Link to PMDD Identified: An Expert Interview With David R. Rubinow, MD. Author: David R. Rubinow, MD

[73] Parkinson's Disease Information Page from NIH Neurological Institute

[74] Psychology Today. Emily Deans M.D. Iron, Dopamine, and ADHD. Iron influences brain maturation and deficiency may play a role in ADHD. 2015.

dopamine and norepinephrine in the brain, as well as helping keep more dopamine in the synapse.

All of these conditions could benefit from research done on D-MER because a better understanding of D-MER could bring a better understanding of dopamine. Most of the issues above have inappropriate dopamine activity that is either constant or unpredictable and thus very hard to predict or measure. Mothers with D-MER however have a very reliable and predictable response that could be useful in the medical community for further research and understanding about dopamine and its normal vs. abnormal activity.

It is important to point out that there have been no predispositions or correlations shown between other dopamine related conditions and D-MER. Just because a mother has D-MER, there is currently nothing to suggest that she is at risk for other dopamine mediated health conditions.

Why Research Is Not Being Done
With all the benefits of learning more and with all the questions that need to be answered, it is normal for many mothers to be baffled as to why formal research is not being conducted. There are likely many answers and reasons for this and some of the more evident ones can be deduced.

There is still a limited knowledge about dopamine. Dopamine is still vastly mysterious in many ways and a lot of studies are being published on a regular basis to gain further insight on it. It is true that D-MER could add answers about dopamine where some conditions still remain opaque with regards to the involvement of dopamine. However, as Parkinson's Disease is widely spread and debilitating, D-MER is not, and thus, the efforts to understand dopamine are present, just not in relation to D-MER at this time.

D-MER now has a large group of self-selected mothers. Though it is wonderful that mothers have found help, answers and community, it does actually also make some kinds of research more difficult. Self-selection bias arises any time in which people select themselves into a group, causing a biased sample with what is called: non-probability sampling. To find mothers that could participate in a study that have not already classified themselves as having D-MER would prove difficult. Additionally, self-selected communities quickly begin to have a shared understanding and explanations of their experience, which are often not based on stringent scientific research.

It is possible to find interested scientists for D-MER research, but it simply has not happened yet. Currently, no organized task force exists that brings the issue of D-MER to organizations like the National Health Institute. There are facilities that have grants for research but either a researcher has to take interest in D-MER of their own accord, or the topic needs to be introduced to the right researcher.

For some researchers D-MER may be met with skepticism and/or a lack of urgency. Those that experience D-MER have a true sense of passion for learning and discovering more about D-MER, but it is possible that to the research community, it is difficult to find a robust argument to justify spending time and resources into research on this topic. This might be due to the view that not enough individuals are affected by D-MER, that it appears to run it's course naturally, and that the experiences are not of urgent enough nature.

The kinds of research that are viable in the medical community are few and complicated. Viable studies include: meta-analysis, systematic review, randomized controlled trial, cohort study (prospective observational study), case-control study, cross-sectional study, qualitative studies, case reports and series and ideas, editorials, and opinions. For D-MER right now the easiest of access are case studies (of which there have been three), qualitative studies and reviews, and editorials in medical journals. Other types of study require many more resources, people, expense and a way around the self-selection problem; not to mention the credentials required for publication.

It is unfortunate that more understanding about D-MER cannot be given to the mothers that struggle with it. Many mothers have found help, support and relief from the information and awareness that is currently available. However, this work is far from complete, as much of it is speculation. Mothers who take comfort in the information that they do have, still express frustration over not having more information or answers. Mothers still want to know if they can prevent it, fix it, understand it better, find validation for it, if it puts them at risk for future problems, what caused it, who else has it and many more unanswerable curiosities. Hopefully the future of D-MER will provide some, if not all, of these answers.

Conclusion

It is difficult to compose a conclusion for an issue that remains so far from concluded. As the recognized expert on D-MER I struggle with the fact that I have to answer so much correspondence peppered with language such as, "it seems", "it appears", "D-MER suggests that" and other circumspect terminology. When I write and speak about D-MER, I am unable to do so from an evidence based perspective but I also have to give a voice to all the mothers I have heard from and hope science comes along to back us all up. I hope that it will not be long before I am compelled to write a second edition of this book due to all the new research and evidence being produced about D-MER. Until that time though, mothers with D-MER cannot continue to wait; knowing the validity of their experience and not having anything but sparse amounts of online information available to them, which is why I have attempted to offer the information here.

The most heartbreaking correspondence I get from mothers is from those that have been dismissed and invalidated by their health care providers and this is something that must start shifting. My hope is that the information in this book will help bring more education to care providers so that mothers can find the support that they need to continue nursing. Mothers with D-MER are very susceptible to the dismissal of their experience, as they often start by feeling half way crazy and very uncertain themselves to begin with. A mother with D-MER is much less likely to wean prematurely if she has the support and validation of those around her. I moderate the largest support group for D-MER online and I have never seen such a constantly active group that needs no real moderation. These mothers are posting daily and continually support each other with kindness and encouragement, regardless of their experience, choices or the level of vulnerability shown. As an IBCLC I have never seen a breastfeeding issue that seems to leave mothers so hungry for constant and consistent connection with other mothers struggling with the same issue. Mothers with D-MER continue to feel isolated in their situation and connecting with other mothers with D-MER online is one thing that keeps them feeling not only like they are not isolated, but also that they are normal.

Every mother with D-MER started out feeling like she was a freak, but someday this will not be the case as information continues to spread. In the meantime I write this book to tell you, the mother, you are beautifully normal and your struggle is real. To the healthcare provider I say, the mother you are working with just wants to feel normal and is in desperate need of your support and validation because her struggle is oh so very real.

Resources

- The official website for D-MER
- Follow the latest information about D-MER on Alia Macrina's Facebook page for D-MER
- Talk with other mothers who experience D-MER on the support group page for D-MER on Facebook

- Contact d-mer.org at info@d-mer.org for lactation consulting services about D-MER
- Refer your health care providers to the following published information about D-MER: Link for D-MER on Google Books and Link for D-MER on Google Scholar
- Handouts about D-MER can be download online.
- Find an International Board Certified Lactation Consultant online.
- List Of Books That Reference D-MER

    The Nursing Mother's Companion - Page 171

    The Womanly Art of Breastfeeding: Completely Revised and Updated 8th Edition - Page 416

    Experienced Doula: Advanced Skills for Hospital Doulas - Page 136

    Breastfeeding E-Book: A Guide for the Medical Professional - Page 626

    Breastfeeding and Human Lactation - Page 291

    What to Expect When You're Expecting - Page 616

    Breastfeeding: A Guide for the Medical Profession - Page 606

    Supported in Breastfeeding: Stories of Nourishing Wisdom - Page 74

    The Informed Parent: A Science-Based Resource for Your Child's First Four Years - Page 143

    Mothering Through the Darkness: Women Open Up About the Postpartum Experience

    Parenting, Uncensored: Straight Talk from Real Moms on Breastfeeding

    The Developing Person Through the Life Span

    Breastfeeding Answers Made Simple

    Another Twinkle in the Eye: Contemplating Another Pregnancy After Perinatal Loss

About The Author

Alia's passion is to alert and enlighten women and the breastfeeding community about Dysphoric Milk Ejection Reflex (D-MER) and to encourage further research into this phenomenon.

Though she is an International Board Certified Lactation Consultant (IBCLC), she is also someone who has experienced D-MER firsthand.

Her research of D-MER started in 2007, and was the result of her own experience nursing her third child. She has been dubbed the person "who spoke until somebody listened", because she was not satisfied with the answers that she was receiving from professionals. She states, "I knew that I was unique, but I also knew that I could not be alone in my experience with letdown; I am not THAT special". Since then, D-MER has gained attention in medical and breastfeeding communities worldwide.

As an author, speaker and investigator on the subject of D-MER, she supports mothers and healthcare professionals in the US and internationally, in relation to D-MER. She is in private practice as a lactation consultant in the Finger Lakes region of New York State, and is part of the second generation of lactation consultants who are shining new light inside the field and science of lactation.

In her personal and family life, she is nearing the early part of mid-life as a contentedly divorced and single mother of three home educated children ages 10, 13 and 16. She lives in the often cold, but beautiful Finger Lakes region of western New York state in a small and friendly community of a tiny town that she adores. She resides on an off-the-beaten-path bit of land, and enjoys a simplistic and somewhat organic and natural way of life with her children, along with her two cats and a house trained rabbit.

Dedications and Acknowledgments

This book and this information would not be possible with out two people. Without them this knowledge would not be known as it is today; my mentor and colleague, Diane Wiessinger, and my "D-MER baby", my third and youngest child, Elliotte. My D-MER experience was painful, but the journey has been amazing. So I want to recognize them both in detail.

Thank you to my little baby girl, for seeing us through all of this. You were my perfect home birthed baby, with whom I expected to also have a perfect breastfeeding experience and relationship with. You will never fully understand the impact that breastfeeding you had on the field of lactation. I sometimes feel like I missed out on the most important times of your first years of life. I spent so much of our breastfeeding time in a state of D-MER, loving you every minute of it, but doing my best to pretend you were not even there. It was not fair. To either of us. It was not what I wanted for you and it was not what I wanted, planned or expected for us. But we persevered through that seemingly never ending battle of emotional warfare and we made it through together.

Thank you to wonderful, wonderful Diane. She never minded that I used her at times for her name and status in order to get answers from the better known professionals. She never doubted me even when at times I doubted myself. She countless times talked me away from "the ledge" when I was ready to give up or blow a gasket out of general frustration or discouragement. She poured her emotion into my experience, resonating with my pain and celebrating with me when it was lifted. She used her amazing counseling skills every minute of the way. She herself has poured hundreds of hours into D-MER and it's greater cause and humbly continues to try and give me all the "credit" for the work that has been done, even though without her, it never would have come this far.

Thank you for the kindness and openness of all the mothers with D-MER that I have come across and that remain supportive, engaged and active on the D-MER support group page. All of your voices make a difference every day.

I want to thank my family of choice, who, on the most basic level, supported me and propelled me into continuing on my journey of working within the field of lactation and support of breastfeeding mothers. But on the larger scale, were present in my life these last few years in such a way that I never had room to question or doubt my own ability, strength or worth:

I appreciate the love and commitment of Jeremy Griffith, Nona Ammering, Shane Ammering, Melinda Linz and Matthew Ingraham.

Specifically, I would not be where or who I am with out the impact, support and influence of Brad Johnson, Meredith Perrin, Jharid Minor, Alexandra Wilkosz.

Additionally, I want to express my gratitude for the continued devotion and commitment of Zachary Davis, Bridget Milliman, Susan Oakes Hauf, Nathan R Smith and Jana Wachsler

Lastly, a most special thanks to the longevity and dedication of my closest and most intimate supporter, friend and adviser, Marcelina Watkinson.

And hugs to my biggest babies, Felicia and Noah, who continue to teach me everyday and, by simply being born, helped me figure out what I wanted to be when I grew up.

Figures

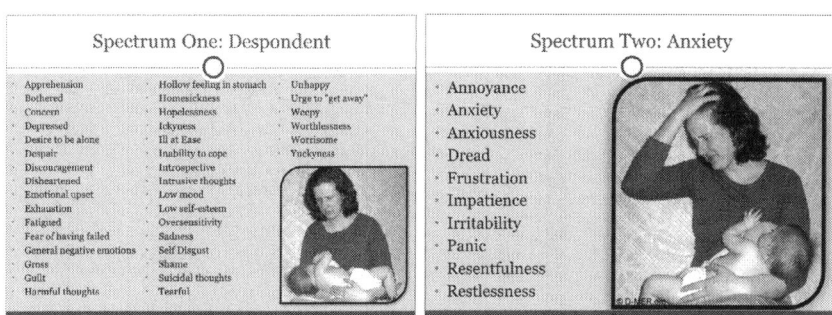

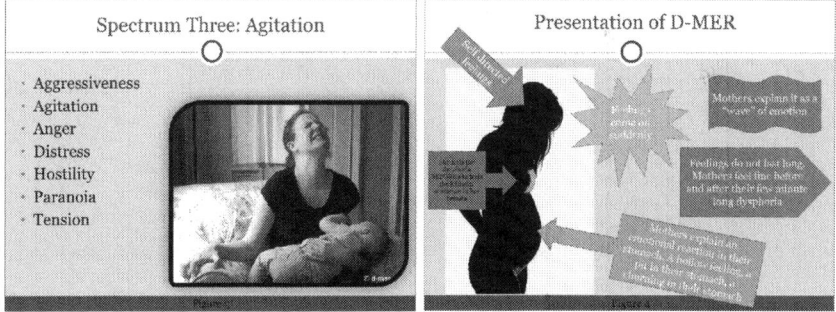

The Intensity in the Spectrum

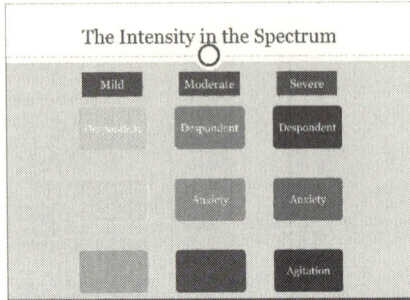

	Mild	Moderate	Severe
Despondent	Despondent	Despondent	Despondent
		Anxiety	Anxiety
			Agitation

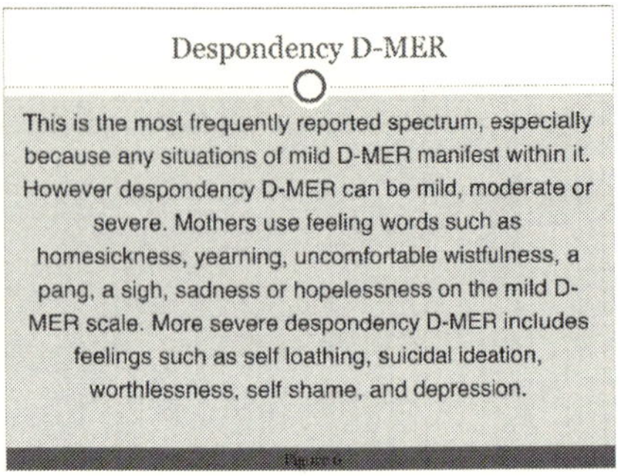

Figure 5

Despondency D-MER

This is the most frequently reported spectrum, especially because any situations of mild D-MER manifest within it. However despondency D-MER can be mild, moderate or severe. Mothers use feeling words such as homesickness, yearning, uncomfortable wistfulness, a pang, a sigh, sadness or hopelessness on the mild D-MER scale. More severe despondency D-MER includes feelings such as self loathing, suicidal ideation, worthlessness, self shame, and depression.

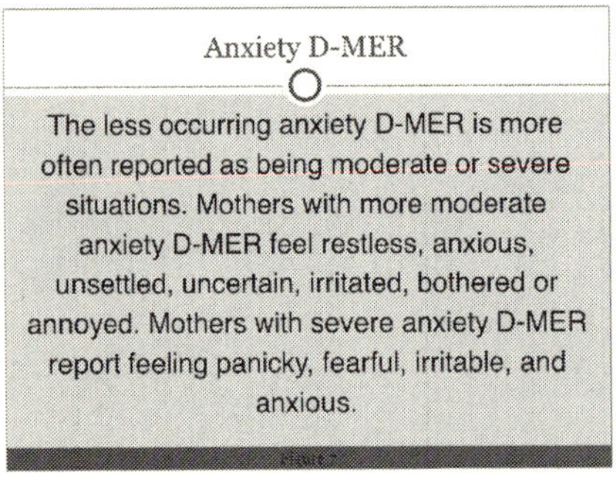

Figure 6

Anxiety D-MER

The less occurring anxiety D-MER is more often reported as being moderate or severe situations. Mothers with more moderate anxiety D-MER feel restless, anxious, unsettled, uncertain, irritated, bothered or annoyed. Mothers with severe anxiety D-MER report feeling panicky, fearful, irritable, and anxious.

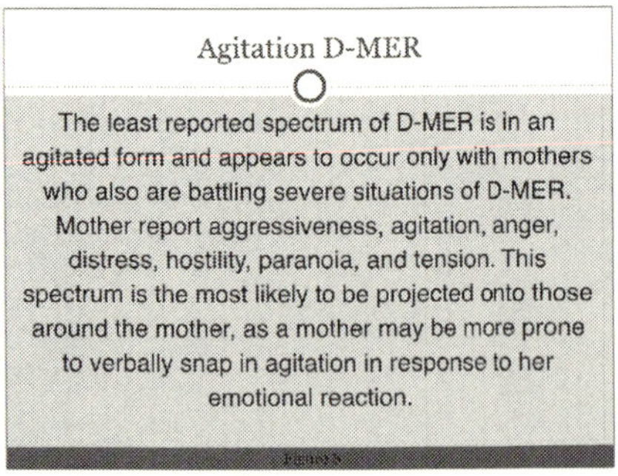

Figure 7

Agitation D-MER

The least reported spectrum of D-MER is in an agitated form and appears to occur only with mothers who also are battling severe situations of D-MER. Mother report aggressiveness, agitation, anger, distress, hostility, paranoia, and tension. This spectrum is the most likely to be projected onto those around the mother, as a mother may be more prone to verbally snap in agitation in response to her emotional reaction.

Figure 8

Mild D-MER

Mild D-MER is often described as a "pang" or a "sigh." A mother takes comfort in knowing her feelings are unjustified but does generally not inquire about treatment. It is often rated in severity on a scale of 1-3 before knowing that D-MER is to blame, and a mother seems to get past feelings nearly all together after education of D-MER. Mild D-MER seems to self correct within the first three months. It often seems to fall on despondency spectrum.

Moderate D-MER

With moderate D-MER a mother rates on a scale of 4-7 before knowing D-MER is the cause. Often the mother lowers her rating to a 2-5 after learning about D-MER. Mothers sometimes show interest in homeopathic or natural remedies. Committed mothers do not seem to waver in their determination to breastfeed through it. Moderate D-MER seems to self correct between 3-9 months. It can fall on all three spectrums, though often leans to the despondency and anxiety spectrums.

Severe D-MER

A mother with severe D-MER rates it on a scale of 7-10 before and after learning about D-MER. Mothers are more likely to wean, despite commitment to even extended breastfeeding. Often D-MER presents with suicidal ideation and other thoughts of self harm. Severe cases seem to not self correct within the first year. It can fall on all three spectrums.

Intensities

Mild

Moderate
- Usually will self correct between 3-9 months
- Some what bothersome to mothers even after education as treatment.
- Some risk to shorter duration of nursing.
- Is usually despondency or anxiety D-MER

Severe

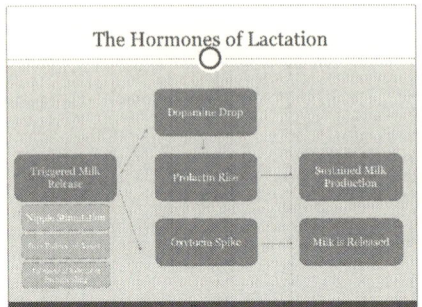

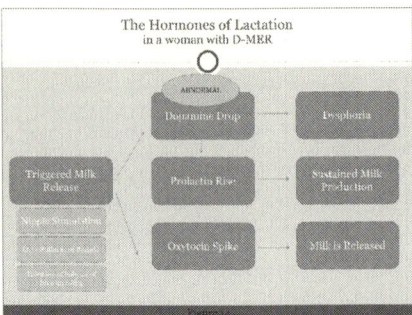

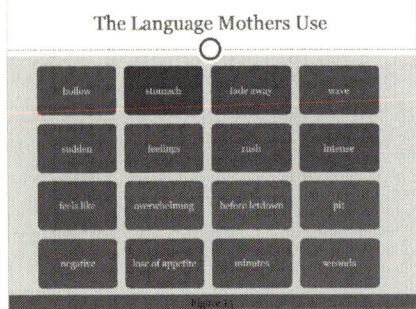

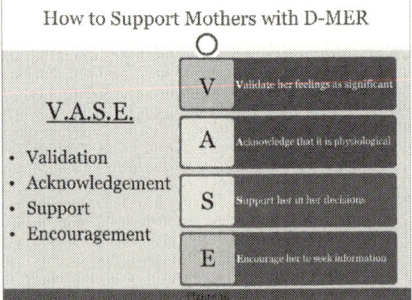

Examples of Mother's Weaning Thresholds

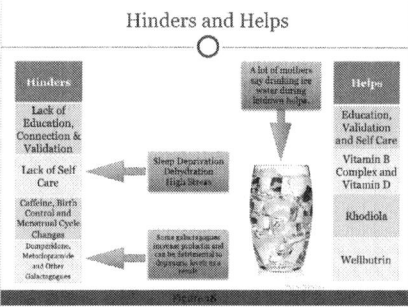

Hinders and Helps

Hinders
- Lack of Education, Connection & Validation
- Lack of Self Care
- Caffeine, Birth Control and Menstrual Cycle Changes
- Domperidone, Metoclopramide and Other Galactogogues

Helps
- Education, Validation and Self Care
- Vitamin B Complex and Vitamin D
- Rhodiola
- Wellbutrin

Thoughts and Feelings of D-MER

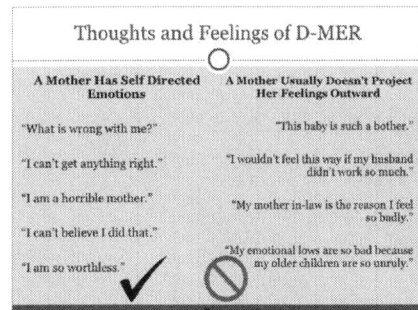

A Mother Has Self Directed Emotions	A Mother Usually Doesn't Project Her Feelings Outward
"What is wrong with me?"	"This baby is such a bother."
"I can't get anything right."	"I wouldn't feel this way if my husband didn't work so much."
"I am a horrible mother."	"My mother in-law is the reason I feel so badly."
"I can't believe I did that."	"My emotional lows are so bad because my older children are so unruly."
"I am so worthless."	

Identifying Mothers With D-MER

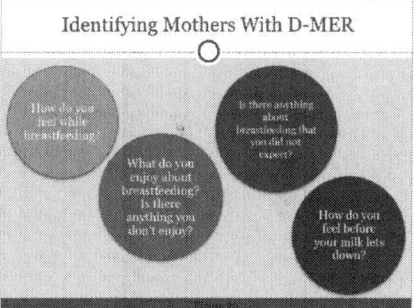

201

Table Of Acronyms

Acronym	Meaning
D-MER	dysphoric milk ejection reflex
CLC	certified lactation consultant
PPD	postpartum depression
LC	lactation consultant
MER	milk ejection reflex
PIF	prolactin inhibiting factor
PIH	prolactin inhibiting hormone
RLS	restless leg syndrome
PCD	post coital dysphoria
SSRI	selective serotonin reuptake inhibitor
PTSD	post traumatic stress disorder
HSP	highly sensitive person
D&C	dilation and curettage
PD	parkinson's disease
IBCLC	international board certified lactation consultant
MOAI	monoamine oxidase inhibitor
EPO	evening primrose oil
CBT	cognitive behavioral therapy
PMDD	premenstrual dysphoric disorder
ADHD	attention deficit hyperactivity disorder

Made in the USA
Middletown, DE
13 September 2019